TRADITIONAL HOME AND HERBAL REMEDIES
BY APPOINTMENT ONLY

J AN DE VRIES'S interest in herbs and natural remedies was first aroused when, as a child during World War II, he was shown the secrets of the herb garden by an old monk in occupied Holland. After training as a pharmacist as an adult, he felt increasingly drawn to this ancient knowledge and learned all he could from Dr Alfred Vogel, the renowned Swiss herbalist; from a group of gypsies who took him up into the mountains; and much later, during his travels in China and the Far East.

Today, more and more people are beginning to rediscover the healing powers of roots and plants, with the help of Jan de Vries and other pioneers in alternative medicine. Indeed, some of the most frequently prescribed and powerful drugs are based on plant extracts.

Jan de Vries has researched as far back as the twelfth century and has recorded the folk wisdom of many of the old people he has met on his travels, learning from them the popular remedies which had been passed on to them by their forefathers.

In *Traditional Home and Herbal Remedies*, the third book in his "By Appointment Only" series Jan de Vries shares with his readers some of these remedies. Everyone who holds his philosophy that nature has a way to help every illness will find this book an invaluable source of information and encouragement.

Traditional Home
and
Herbal Remedies

by

JAN DE VRIES

Introduction by Dr Alfred Vogel
Author of 'The Nature Doctor'

HERBAL MEDICINE/HERBS/ROOTS/SEEDS/BERRIES AND
CURRANTS/VEGETABLES/FRUITS/SEASONINGS/
CEREALS/HOME REMEDIES

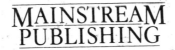

MAINSTREAM
PUBLISHING

First published in 1986, reprinted 1987, by
MAINSTREAM PUBLISHING COMPANY (EDINBURGH) LTD.
7 Albany Street
Edinburgh EH1 3UG

ISBN 1 85158 011 5 (cloth)
ISBN 1 85158 012 3 (Paperback)

Typeset in 11/12 Andover by Mainstream Publishing.
Printed in Great Britain by Collins, Glasgow.

Contents

Books available from the same author in the
By Appointment Only series:

Stress and Nervous Disorders

Multiple Sclerosis

Introduction

IT WAS A fortunate occasion when I met Jan de Vries in January 1959 in The Netherlands. With pleasure and conviction I spoke of my forty years' experience in the field of herbal medicine and my views on diet and nourishment. I soon realised that I had an extremely interested listener who fully appreciated my acquired knowledge of the whole sphere of medical science.

Jan de Vries was not only interested to learn everything about my experiences of when, where and how to collect herbs and which methods were to be followed, he also insisted on taking part in the actual process of extracting beneficial ingredients. As he was a trained and qualified pharmacist, he was already familiar with the world of plants and herbs and had considerable knowledge in this field. He accepted an invitation to join our firm which gave us the chance to establish a working relationship which has lasted for years. He was one of my best pupils, if not the very best, and he had the opportunity to further develop his given talents in the field of natural medicine.

I was very happy to share with him my enthusiasm for

nature and the world of plants, as originated by the sovereign power of the Creator. He was also prepared to accept my principle that herbal medicine should always have priority in the treatment of illnesses.

As a result of our experiences we both agreed that through knowledge and advice on natural methods and herbal remedies it was possible to improve one's health and keep illnesses at bay. Nature itself is capable of healing.

Drawing on my many years of experience I was able to convince Jan de Vries completely that herbal medicine in combination with a natural diet could create positive responses in the body in order to ward off ailments. By creating the right conditions for the body and supplying it with the correct nourishment, one is able to activate one's own regeneration system. In this way it it possible to overcome as well as cure ailments. We realise more and more, and my experience over many years in practice has contributed to this, that we don't just have an important role to play in the curing of illnesses, but also in the prevention of medical disturbances. This requires us to put emphasis on preventive medicine. Prevention is better than a cure.

This principle plays a major role in our programme. In an effort to clarify this to patients and other interested parties, I myself have written several books, such as *The Nature Doctor*, *The Liver as the Regulator of our Health*, and *Nature, Your Guide to Healthier Living*.

Jan de Vries was immediately prepared to share with his friends and later with his patients my experiences and he recommended these books for their information. He is, I am pleased to repeat, my most successful "pupil". His success from which many patients have benefited is, however, not only a result of his talents, it is also thanks to the Creator who has supplied so many plants with healing powers.

INTRODUCTION

I am very pleased that Jan de Vries is making the effort of sharing his knowledge and experiences with us on paper. His books are written in a simple language, readily understood by both patients and laymen alike. In them he deals with natural ways and methods using herbal remedies to overcome ailments and illnesses.

It is important that not just the obvious symptoms are cured as conventional medicine would teach us. We must look for the cause of the illness in order to continue the treatment and find a cure for the source. Very little benefit is obtained by clearing up an ache or easing a sensitivity if we are not able to eliminate the cause. In order to do this we should study the whole person and attempt to recognise which factors have contributed to this condition. There could be very many reasons — for example, a breathing difficulty or a movement disorder, shortage of oxygen, rest or sleep. There can be so many causes of a biological imbalance.

Jan de Vries has acquired and developed a large knowledge in this area. With perseverance he builds up an overall picture of total health, not forgetting the physical and mental conditions of the patient.

I am convinced that in this book he will show many sufferers the right way to recovery in plain and simple language. It is an excellent complement to my books, as we have both sincerely attempted to serve our fellow men and share with them our knowledge acquired from our understanding and experience of the bounty of nature.

Dr Alfred Vogel

11

1

Herbal Medicine

DURING A visit in 1984 with a group of well-known professors, doctors, homoeopaths, herbalists and other alternative practitioners, to the Karolinska Institute in Stockholm — an institute, incidentally, that has the oldest medical library in the world — I was most impressed when Dr Voll and I were shown a special book. It was one of the oldest volumes in medical history, containing a collection of views which we see gaining ground again today. In that old book we discovered great amounts of valuable advice which is still applicable today. It all goes back to God's promise at the creation: "That there be herbs for healing".

Browsing through this medical library and looking into the medical history prior to the establishment of homoeopathy, we saw remedies in books which are being used to great effect today. Looking at it, we can be grateful that in this day and age so much of ancient medical knowledge has been rediscovered. After all, if perhaps a fraction of all the money which is spent in medical research today had been spent to research God's natural healing gifts to mankind, I am sure that we would have gained a lot of knowledge. Weren't even the healing properties of Digitalis or Foxglove found by accident? And haven't they been a blessing to millions of people?

I was greatly surprised when Dr Vogel and I took a group of medical students into the Jura Hills and showed them weeds, herbs and roots, which were growing there and of which the students had no knowledge. My dear old friend, Dr Vogel, who has given his lifetime to the study of herbs and plants used medicinally and has been a blessing to so many people, told this group about some of the purposes of these horticultural gifts over which we often tread without realisation of their healing powers.

I remember very well as a child that a very old herbalist lived in our town. Many people went to him and even though his knowledge of the healing properties was limited, he was in great demand. I also used to sit at my grandmother's feet and listen to her wonderful stories about the gifts with which Mother Nature had supplied us. Her knowledge had been passed down from her mother and some of these old treatments we can see back in use today.

It is a really wonderful thing to think that in our lifetime some of these marvellous remedies are again getting the attention they deserve.

I have been practising in Scotland for over fifteen years. If we look back over the history of medicine even as far back as the thirteenth century, many of the beautiful abbeys in Jedburgh, Kelso, Melrose, Dryburgh, Newbattle, Holyrood, Kilwinning and even Culzean Castle had herb gardens. Everywhere we find here the learning of what was given by nature to alleviate human suffering. Each monastery or priory had translations of ancient medical books in which herbs used by the monks were described. Medicinal plants include the rose, the bean, the savoury, the cummin, the fennel, the lily, the sage, the mint, etc, etc.

There is a huge variety of wonderful plants, herbs and roots which were used then and are in use once again today. If I think however of the treasures of horticulture which have not yet been researched and the knowledge we might still gather then that research will be more than worth while.

I fully realised this during a visit to South Africa when in the Cape Province I was shown some herbal plants which had never been researched before, till an old professor, anxious to learn more about them, conducted some experiments with the plants. One of these plants today is being used for cancer treatment.

Time and time again we are left to stand in wonder and amazement by the life energy contained by some plants, roots and herbs.

If we look deep into the resources of the British Museum in London, where Britain's oldest and most precious manuscripts are kept, we see writings compiled over centuries. We are again surprised by the wonderful healing methods which were used by our forefathers, whose knowledge we have inherited through these manuscripts. Few people are aware of the existence of these books, let alone have had the opportunity to study them, but the knowledge we can gain here is considerable. They give us an insight into the medical history of Britain over the centuries and describe many natural healing methods which once more are gaining popularity.

Varieties of herbal potions have often unjustly been referred to as placebos. Nowadays, though, we know that herbal potions have been of assistance to many people. The magical workings of extracts and mixtures have been used for centuries to the benefit of mankind. Much is written about these simple, harmless and generally useful remedies. Even the *Primitive Physic* or *The Easy and Natural Method of Curing Most Diseases* composed by John Wesley

TRADITIONAL HOME AND HERBAL REMEDIES

(1703-1791) had reached its 21st edition by 1785. All these writings, including today's publications, give us an insight into the traditions of old folk medicine.

I would like to take you for a little walk in the kingdom of herbs, plants and roots and all that grows in God's nature. I will pick a few leaves, pull a few herbs, look at a few weeds and tell you why over the years they have been of such help in my practice.

Some traditional British, especially Scottish, herbs have been used throughout history as home remedies. I not only marvel at their efficacy and suitability for so many purposes, but am also surprised at their multitude. It has been a pleasure to me that not only my old gardener, who has been so loyal to me over the years, but also a doctor's widow from South Uist as well as many other people have given me information. I feel privileged that so many patients have shared with me some of these old methods and cures which have been handed down for generations by their forefathers and it is my sincere hope that the reader of this book will get the same pleasure and benefit.

Over the twenty-five years that I have been in practice, thousands of testimonials from all over the world have reached me. If ever I were asked if I believe that there are plants, herbs and roots to cure every illness, my honest answer must be: YES.

The effects of the medicinal properties of that which grows in the soil is the way to good health. Many people, having gone through the conventional channels of doctors and hospitals have come to me and I have turned to nature for advice. They have been able to regain their health, having found an answer to the hopelessness of suffering, with the aid of some perhaps old but not forgotten methods.

2

Herbs

IT IS NO more than a year ago that I discovered from my
mother's side I am descended from a long line of families
which practised herbal medicine. As a child I was always
intrigued by the stories my grandmother told regarding
this particular subject, but what I did not know was that
her mother's family in Germany came from a long line of
herbalists. So when as a child my grandmother taught me
her love of nature, I used to go into the fields finding the
different herbs which possessed healing powers. This
feeling got stronger when I worked in Switzerland and I
went up into the mountains with the gypsies, who have
taught me more about herbal medicine than anybody else.

I clearly remember a period during the Second World
War when my mother was asked to help out in the badly hit
area around Arnhem. The house where she was based was
next to a monastery and I got to know an old monk there in
charge of the herbal garden, who taught me some of his
knowledge.

The first herb I learnt about was the marigold. I looked at
this flower whose Latin name is *Calendula Officinalis* and

learnt that it was used by the Romans on the first day of every month. I did not know it then, but found out later that Calendula is a wonderful remedy to aid the healing of wounds. The monk also told me that the old alchemists would chase away evil spirits with the Calendula. With all his interesting stories he aroused something in me and my interest in the field of herbal medicine has never waned.

The monk also told me about the Shepherd's Purse (*Capsella Bursa Pastoris*) and though I was not aware then, nowadays Shepherd's Purse is used as an effective remedy for internal bleedings and also for menstrual problems.

He showed me the *Centaurium Umbellatum* — our cornflower — and told me that the old Greeks used this plant for stomach problems and to improve the appetite. However, in our modern society Centaurium is a wonderful remedy for the problem of Anorexia Nervosa.

I could go on, but in this book I will mention some of the remedies I prescribe quite often and which have become the mainstay of my practice.

It is fascinating when we look at herbs today, to realise the link they give us with the ancient civilisations of China, Greece, Egypt and India — countries where I have looked at herbs and found the herbs of modern day are the same as we read about in the Bible or even in the Sumerian tablets 2000 BC.

The practical use of herbs or plants for either culinary or medicinal purposes will give the reader an idea of how much can be done to alleviate suffering through the use of these harmless remedies. A good herbalist is merely concerned with the question of why the body has not been able to heal itself. He will try to direct and influence the vital force or the life energy with the help of herbs and plants to overcome the problem.

The majority of illnesses can be cured by herbalism, which can also be used as a prevention of disease. When I travelled to China, where I worked for a period of time, I learnt to combine traditional and preventive medicine. These methods combine well together and preventive health care is so important because of the way our bodies are under attack in these modern times. It is of the utmost importance that we keep the vital force of the plant as unadulterated as possible. One of the reasons I like Dr Vogel's preparations is that when I studied with him I witnessed that he only used fresh herbs and plants. Their juices were extracted and conserved so that the obtained product was as fresh as possible. He is almost the only person in the world who manages to do this.

It is impossible to always explain the exact workings of those plants and herbs created by God. The well-known Emil Schlegel stated that each blossom which blooms in the garden and each leaf which grows, speaks a mystic language. We then realise that today in this busy life of ours there are things we just cannot explain and that are beyond human understanding, but which we have to accept as gifts to help mankind. We have to respect this healing power. A well-known Dutch poet puts it beautifully:

> my spreekt de blomme 'n taele
> my is't cruydt beleeft
> my is't altemaele
> wat God gheschaepen heeft

This simply means that all is given to us, free and for nothing, because it is created for us and it speaks a language which only the understanding heart can recognise.

Echinacea Purpurea Herba

Dr Vogel was once interviewed for a popular magazine

together with a Professor of Medicine. They were both asked what they would prescribe as an antibiotic. The Professor of Medicine answered that he had 300 to 400 drugs to choose from. Dr Vogel's answer was that the medicine he most often prescribed was a herbal remedy called Echinaforce. This is derived from the *Echinacea Purpurea Herba* with its attractive pink flower. A fresh herbal preparation suitable for many purposes is obtained.

This remedy has indeed been a blessing to numerous people. The herb is not found a great deal in this country, although it could grow well enough in Britain. The plant and flower originates from Mexico, where it is used in the treatment of infections and inflammations.

Echinaforce, made of 95% *Echinacea Purpurea Herba* and 5% *Echinacea Purpurea Radix* into a fresh herb preparation, can be used as a non-specific therapy. In Germany and Switzerland it has become very popular and today it is known as one of the finest natural antibiotics. Echinaforce causes an increase in the body's resistance against colds and it is suitable in cases of dermatological problems. Internally it clears septic processes and the processes of inflammation, giving a faster healing effect.

After working with this particular remedy for nearly twenty-five years, I was not surprised that Dr Vogel singled out the preparation for mention in the interview, because even today I am still amazed at the results my patients receive from the use of Echinaforce.

I would like to share a few of my experiences concerning this effective natural antibiotic with you.

One day, a young couple, who are both doctors, contacted me. They had tried unsuccessfully for a baby and asked me for some advice. After a period of time I received a card bearing the news that a baby girl had been born, to everyone's delight. Not long after the birth of the baby, however, the father phoned me in despair and told me that the baby was in hospital where numerous antibiotics had been tried, but that the baby's constant diarrhoea could not be stopped. He was desperate and asked if I could perhaps think of something which could be of help. I told him about Albert Schweitzer who treated so many people in Lamborene successfully with the Echinacea extract. I also told him that if he phoned Dr Vogel, he would immediately be told to use Echinaforce and I reminded him that we had discussed this remedy before and that I had experienced occasions where everything else had failed and yet Echinaforce had brought results.

I instructed him to start carefully with five drops, three times a day and then step it up a little. After a week he phoned me to say that to his delight the remedy had worked and that his daughter was saved. Proof again indeed of what a wonderful remedy this is.

A patient comes to mind who lives close to my clinic and who had a dermatological problem which I diagnosed after a few tests as being a wheat allergy. Even after banning wheat from her diet, the problem persisted and she despaired. I prescribed a massive dose of Echinaforce: three times daily 30 drops and within ten days the problem was cleared. How grateful she was.

I would like to mention a few more first-hand experiences with this remedy which I always carry with me wherever I travel throughout the world. Once I had practised all day in my clinic in Preston, Lancashire, and at the end, being a little tired, one of my patients unfortunately sneezed straight into my face. I went out and washed my face thoroughly with disinfectant, but the next day my jaws were swollen and very sore. I decided to see my dentist, who is also a good friend of mine. When he saw the situation he told me there and then: "Jan, if you don't immediately take a strong antibiotic you are going to lose all your teeth." This was a shock to me, because I took pride in the fact that I still had all my own teeth and I was nearly tempted to take his advice.

He knew my principles on the subject of drugs, so I told him that I would try Echinaforce first. He laughed at me and told me that I would never be able to do it. I asked him for a prescription just in case I failed with Echinaforce, which I would try for one day. I would then accept his advice and take the prescribed antibiotic. I went home and took 4 X daily 30 drops of Echinaforce and by the next day I had overcome the crisis. It was with pride and relief that I went to see my dentist to return the prescription. He was utterly amazed and since then he has advised people to use Echinaforce. It is indeed a most remarkable remedy which still manages to surprise me at times.

Another personal experience I had with Echinaforce was not long ago when I was suffering from a cold. Usually I shake this off pretty quickly, but unfortunately I had to travel abroad at the time. When I stepped off the plane I knew that some of the catarrh had lodged itself in my left ear. Whatever I did, I became almost deaf in the left ear and nothing seemed to shift the catarrh. For several weeks I tried to overcome this deafness to no avail and I decided at long last to use quite a heavy dose of Echinaforce, which cleared the catarrhal condition so that I fully regained my hearing.

Very often with patients, when normal remedies for a particular condition are prescribed and do not bring relief, I introduce this remedy as an extra reserve or back-up to help people. As for people who travel to sunny, hot countries and are susceptible to infections or inflammations, I always advise them to carry the remedy in their suitcase.

Often when I lecture at medical meetings or seminars I mention this plant with its marvellous healing powers. It ought to be used widely and if only more credence was given to it, a greater choice of non-drug treatments would become available.

When I see the results of these remedies it makes me think of an old testament quotation. In the book of Ecclesiastes it says that the Lord has created medicines out of the earth and he that is wise will not abhor them.

Marigold – Calendula officinalis

This remedy again is widely used in my clinic. Calendula is one of our native herbs which is known in Britain for its healing powers. In the old folk medicine books we read that the plant's flowers, stems and leaves were gathered and used and although the Calendula resembles the *Arnica* it has a different working. As a blood cleanser it is a great help. It stimulates circulation but it also is a wonderful remedy for the healing of wounds.

Calendula ointment in combination with other remedies is recommended in cases of phlebitis, varicose veins, circulatory problems, etc. Calendula ointment is also a wonderful help with athlete's foot and skin problems which are difficult to heal. Even with cancerous sores, ulcers and swellings several of my patients have found Calendula ointment a great help.

The case of a particular lady who unfortunately had a red, spotty nose, comes to mind. She was very often teased about this and felt embarrassed. She had almost reached the stage of an irrecoverable inferiority complex. After having used some homoeopathic remedies, which largely cleared the redness, I advised her to use the Calendula ointment to try to lose the little spots. It was amazing how, slowly but surely, the problem cleared up.

If we cleanse boils or wounds with boiled water added to which are a few drops of marigold tincture, I have found that even varicose ulcers closed. If used in dried form I generally advise patients that the flower, leaves and the stem should be used. Calendula is beneficial for complaints of constipation or swelling of the glands, as well as for stomach pains.

It is interesting to note that according to old folklore it was used in Britain to spice cheese and buns. These were known as marigold buns. Again it gives us an idea of how far we have moved away in our diets from the natural foods and remedies, which have proved their worth in old folk medicine.

If Calendula is combined with distilled water or with witchhazel into a lotion, it makes a soothing combination. The healing powers of this attractive plant are remarkable.

I remember that as a child I used to think that this must be one of the few plants to flourish in my father's garden. When I looked at the golden colour, I often thought that one way or another people must be able to make gold out of this plant. Indeed, in my practice I have found that it has often been as good as gold for many problems where other treatments were not successful.

St John's wort – Hypericum perforatum

The three especially well-known herbs in Britain must be St John's wort (or Rose of Sharon), Goldenrod and Arnica. We don't know how far these herbs go back in history, but I am sure it is much further than we can trace. In history books we read about the colonising armies of Rome and their knowledge of the Mediterranean healing plants. As mentioned previously, herb gardens sprang up in many places during that period.

It is also interesting to see that from the fifteenth century onwards a lot of people used herbal medicine. This practice declined slightly in the sixteenth, seventeenth and eighteenth centuries, and even more so in the early nineteenth century. Although some doctors in the

24

nineteenth century still obtained their medicine from plant sources, it is notable that during that period medical science changed drastically. Through the industrial revolution, which brought more prosperity, the herbalist became more and more a background figure.

In the country, however, and especially in the Highlands of Scotland, certain herbal remedies kept their place. When medical herbalists were refused their status herbal medicine fortunately remained alive in these areas and served a purpose where drugs failed. The picture in my own country, The Netherlands, was similar, but in Germany and Switzerland herbal medicine was kept in high esteem and more research was done there than in any other country.

I still believe that when the thalidomide and other drug scares became public, more awareness of herbal medicine and an interest in alternative medicine was created. We can see a total swing back, as people are becoming aware of the possible side-effects of drugs. I am happy to see that nowadays a healthy balance is developing between orthodox and alternative medicine.

When I considered writing about *Hypericum* or St John's wort, a typical case history came to mind. The patient concerned was a well-known ballet dancer. She had some serious circulatory problems, which showed in cold hands, cold feet, varicose veins, haemorrhoids, etc. She came to me after having gone through a whole range of drugs for these problems prescribed by her own doctor. I put her on a remedy called Hyperisan, which contains *Hypericum perforatum* as one of the four ingredients. Almost within a month the change in this particular lady was noticeable and it was her own doctor who asked with great interest what I had used. I told him that it was sad to see how many people in Scotland were treading over this beautiful flower Hypericum, without realising its medicinal worth.

My patient kept remarkably fresh and young-looking and when she was of advanced age she was interviewed by one of the big papers about her work. She said that she never travels without her bottle of Hyperisan and that she would never forget how much she owed this herb.

I could not begin to tell how helpful Hyperisan has been, not only for circulatory problems, but also as a general tonic. I am reminded of when I started my practice in Scotland and I was not able to get my supplies from Switzerland quickly enough. When I started I was dependent on 25 litres of Hyperisan which I had brought over from The Netherlands. Practically every patient had to be given Hyperisan as a basic tonic, so in that initial period, when I had not much else to start out with, I learned to value its properties.

As well as using this remedy internally for circulatory problems, we can also use it externally as St John's wort oil. The oil together with the drops of the extract proves its worth in phlebitis cases, for example. For bruising or wounds St John's wort oil is invaluable. It is also useful, however, for the young child who has bed-wetting problems, if given in combination with Galeopsis. This is another herbal plant which, if rubbed over the bladder area before going to sleep, has solved many bed-wetting problems of children over the years, just as Hypericum administered internally as well as externally has relieved many mothers suffering from pain in the coccyx while giving birth.

St John's wort in history is very often referred to as "Child from the Sun in Summer". Nowadays we have some marvellous homoeopathic remedies containing St John's wort which are invaluable in the treatment of depressive patients, and even in cases of severe manic depression good results have been obtained.

I remember that my uncle, who worked in a psychiatric

hospital, very often prescribed Hypericum to severely depressed patients and also to those in the closed wards where the more difficult patients were being kept. It was a great calming influence upon them. This is the reason that St John's wort is often called the "Arnica of the Nerves" and, as has already been mentioned, for circulatory problems it is also of particular benefit.

The remedy Hyperisan consists of St John's wort, horse chestnut, yarrow and arnica and has earned its place on the list of valuable herbal remedies. In the olden days people made a tincture or a wine of St John's wort. Through history we see that concoctions were made of the flowers and seeds, to be drunk in wine, which seemed to serve its purpose.

Yarrow – Achillea Millefolium

The next component of Hyperisan is yarrow, known in herbal history under several names, such as millefoile, nosebleed, soldier's herb, bloodwort and woundwort. It is a medicinal herb we could not do without. Yarrow helps with circulatory disorders and vascular spasms. It is also used successfully for angina pectoris and ointments for external use are excellent in the treatment of haemorrhoids and varicose veins.

Yarrow is also used for women with menstrual problems and many a good gynaecologist has prescribed it to regulate the menstrual flow. As a fresh herb preparation used in Hyperisan, it aids the congested blood-flow from all organs. It is often called "the cure of all ills", as it is blood-cleansing and has a blood renewal effect. Yarrow is a herb which does credit to its many names.

Horse Chestnut – Aesculus Hippocastanum

The next component of Hyperisan is the horse chestnut.

TRADITIONAL HOME AND HERBAL REMEDIES

We know that people in the olden days used to carry a horse chestnut in their pocket and believed that by doing so they would be protected from rheumatism.

It is a lesser-known remedy but nevertheless as a tincture is a marvellous help for venous congestion, varicose veins and haemorrhoids. It positively influences and stimulates the general circulation. Gypsies like to feed their horses with chestnuts and Spanish farmers fed them to their cattle to increase the milk productivity. A well-loved tree for its beauty, the tincture made of the horse chestnut forms a valuable component in the remedy Hyperisan.

A letter written by Mme de Sevigne in October 1671 reads: "The other day I had three or four baskets full of chestnuts. Some I boiled, some I roasted and some I put in my pocket." It shows that the properties of the chestnut were known centuries ago.

Mountain Arnica – Arnica Montana

It has always amazed me that over the centuries in The Netherlands, Germany, Switzerland, as well as in Scotland, arnica has never disappeared into the background. Sometimes we call it the herb of the generations and the healing powers of arnica justify any claims.

Arnica Montana — one of the finest herbs — comes up to every expectation. Up in the hills in Switzerland this herb grows richly and is of superb quality. It is very versatile and can be used on minor cuts and grazes.

Arnica, as one of the components of Hyperisan, is used to combat inflammation and aid circulation, and is even helpful in cases of inflammation of the veins which are so difficult to heal. Moreover, patients with high blood pressure or arteriosclerosis may also benefit. A good practitioner knows when to prescribe it and I have often

28

done so to expectant and nursing mothers in order to protect them from varicose veins which often result from pregnancy.

Arnica may be used for traumatic experiences as it has a soothing effect on the nervous system. If suffering from one of the most annoying pains — toothache — a little arnica liquid on a piece of cotton wool placed on the affected tooth will never disappoint.

Frequently with concussions or boils, if arnica ointment is used, it not only produces a soothing but also a healing effect.

Sage – Salvia Officianalis

Sage is yet another well-known herb, grown in Britain and northern Europe, which originated from the Romans. Its lovely name *Salvia* means "health" and it is well known that in the olden days one thought that it was not only physically, but also mentally of great value.

In China it is greatly admired and used, especially by older Chinese who use it to infuse as a tea. They consider it as a great help to the memory.

It is also often used as a mouthwash and for common colds and is beneficial even for stomach problems. The phosphorous content in sage helps the nerves and gives a peaceful sleep. This is largely the reason why ladies with menopausal problems, suffering from excessive perspiration, have achieved remarkable benefits.

A lady who had been through the whole list of orthodox medicine, even using oestrogen, consulted me a while ago. She was still plagued with heavy perspiration. After using sage for a month she came back happily, to tell me that her perspiration problem had disappeared. I advised her to stay on sage for a while longer to make sure that the problem would be solved once and for all.

In old Roman history it was called the secret herb, as

throughout the Middle Ages it was used for many purposes. Father Kneipp said in his writings that no man who owned a garden should forget to plant a head of sage in it.

It is a wonderful name "sage", which means "to save", to cure or to heal. It certainly deserves these names with its many medicinal properties.

Lavender – Lavendula Vera

Lavender must bring back memories to most readers of visits to grandparents. It used to be dried and sewn into little sachets, which were placed in the linen cupboards, where it served a dual purpose: to ward off moths while its delicious scent penetrated the linen.

Lavender is not only a garden attraction, it has been known for centuries as a disinfectant, a tonic and a carminative (medicine to relieve flatulence). Lavender-oil can be used to relieve migraine headaches, digestive disorders and even aid vertigo (dizziness). Infusions of lavender have been of great help as a stimulant or a tonic. It is also beneficial for most bronchial problems.

Mistletoe – Viscum Album

The mistletoe has been the subject of numerous myths and legends. The independent behaviour of this strange, half-parasite plant suggests something very unusual. It needs a tree for its base and its spherical shape makes itself a life on the host tree.

Generations back, physicians like Hippocrates and Dioscorides found the mistletoe a valuable source and today it is used in cancer therapy. In the olden days in Germanic mythology the plant was used by Gallic priests in their religious services. Older generations have woven tales around this evergreen plant.

Father Kneipp advised the use of mistletoe not only for cramps, circulation problems and epileptic fits, but also for cancer. Although mysterious tales have circulated about mistletoe, it is scientifically proven that the plant may be used successfully for problems where other remedies have failed. It is without doubt that it stimulates the cell metabolism in cases of nervous advanced age syndrome. The Druids called it the plant that heals all ills, which sounds like an exaggeration. I have however found in my clinic that where high blood pressure tablets prescribed by the orthodox doctor had no success, *Viscum Album* always proved a useful remedy and this was also true in cases of blood diseases.

As an anti-spasmodic for blood disease problems we have found benefit from this unusual plant as well as in progressed cancer therapy. In the Iscador therapy, with which I have worked for many years, some successes have been beyond expectations where mistletoe has been used.

When I see the mistletoe in so many houses at Christmas, I often wonder if people realise the medicinal values of this wonderful plant. To illustrate its healing powers I relate the experiences of one particular lady who was sent to me with only a few months left to live.

I started her treatment, which was for a disease of the blood, and I prescribed *Viscum Album*. After a while the constant dizziness, which was one of her main complaints, started to improve. The spells of vertigo faded and the pins and needles, which were a constant problem to her, became less bothersome. With mistletoe or *Viscum Album* in combination with a solution derived from the *Petasitus Officianalis* this lady achieved significant results.

Mistletoe has the remarkable characteristic of balancing high and low blood pressure problems. Several research groups have reached the conclusion that mistletoe has a healthy and balancing influence.

TRADITIONAL HOME AND HERBAL REMEDIES

Butterbur – Petasites Officianalis

This particular plant was famous especially in the time of the plague and earned a great reputation in helping to break the fever. People who referred to it in those days claimed that it drove out the pest.

When I think about this plant and how often I have used it over the years, I remember reading the words of the German philosopher Ludwig Feuerbach who once said that in the perishable petals of a flower resides more spirit and life than in the great granite boulder which has had to fight the wear and tear of thousands of years.

Sometimes people say that homoeopathic and nature cures work slowly. I remember a patient who went to his own extremely orthodox doctor and showed him a bottle. He told him that I had prescribed the contents of that bottle for the treatment of his ulcers. The doctor said that he might just as well drink water as the liquid held no medicinal properties. How very untrue. If there is one plant which is entitled to lay claim to such vital spirit and which works directly at the root of the problem, it is the Petasites.

I have used this versatile remedy over the years for a wide variety of problems and it has never let me down. Problems such as spastic conditions, weak circulation, recovery from infections, cases of nutrition deficiencies, ulcers and weakened conditions may all be treated with Petasan. This nice umbrella-like plant has given many people reason for gratitude as Petasan may be used as a replacement for cortisone. Even in cancer therapy we have seen good results with this particular remedy.

I would like to relate a few stories in connection with Petasites. One evening an orthodox doctor brought his wife to me with severe stomach problems. It was diagnosed that she suffered from colitis and diverticulitis, but she had not responded to any treatment and her husband/doctor realised that the diagnosis must be wrong. The latest diagnosis was that she suffered from a dyspepsia problem and I went through several remedies with her which made little change. I then said to the doctor that I felt she should use Petasites, one of the strongest remedies in phytotherapy (that part of medicine that concerns itself with the application of herbal medicine in the case of sick persons). It was amazing but in a few weeks' time her condition already showed considerable improvement and both of them were excited. The doctor insisted on hearing about all the characteristics of this remedy, which he has since prescribed to his own patients.

Tell this story to the doctor who told his patient that he might just as well drink water!

Another story about Petasites concerns a policeman who consulted me a few years ago. This young man was desperate and frustrated as he was unable to carry out his job. This had all started when he was called out to a pub one evening where during a fight someone gave him a knock on the head. He blacked out and was taken to hospital. On his arrival the duty doctor thought that the wounded policeman had had a slight heart attack which was entered in his case history. This was the beginning of his unfortunate story. Because he still had blackouts from time to time he was diagnosed as having minor heart trouble and was declared unfit to work.

This condition had actually lasted for seven years when he finally came to see me. After having looked him over I could really find nothing wrong with his heart or blood pressure. I had however a suspicion that there could be something wrong with his neck. I found it necessary to take a few X-rays and it was then that I became certain that that was the key to most of his problems. I adjusted his third and fourth cervical vertebrae and there was an almost visible relief. However he still suffered spasmodic feelings of dizziness. I then decided to give him *Petasites Officianalis* together with Petadolor, which is a remedy based on Petasites, prescribed for migraines and headaches. At his next visit he reported that the dizziness and blackouts had disappeared and consequently he was able to return to work.

Petasites had again come up to expectations. Its healing powers also manifest themselves in a letter from a cancer patient who had made a miraculous recovery and who wrote: "I thank my Creator that I have met you, but moreover that He has supplied us with such powerful remedies in His nature. I am so grateful to be able to participate again in life and perform my daily duties."

Lily of the Valley – Convallaria Majalis

Lily of the valley is such a delightful flower to look at and in spring it is a feast to the eye. Although its appearance provides such pleasure it also has the marvellous characteristic of stimulating and strengthening the heart.

The lily of the valley goes back to the Middle Ages and was well known even then as a remedy for the heart. When later the more potent, but less safe, Digitalis was discovered, the lily of the valley receded a little into the background. It was however not justified that *Convallaria* disappeared from the scene because certain dangers connected with Digitalis do not exist with lily of the valley. It not only strengthens the heart muscles, but also works as a mild diuretic and in many cases Convallaria has been instrumental in obtaining relief in cases of heart complications, heart or kidney diseases, arteriosclerotic conditions, high blood pressure, premature ageing processes and tachycardia (abnormally fast heartbeat).

One elderly lady who consulted me, told me that

everything had been done to try and control her tachycardia, without producing the desired results. She had decided to come and see me as a last resort. Till this day she still uses Convascillan which is a mixture of Convallaria Majalis, Convallaria juice and Scilla Maritima.

Sometimes it is said that the Convallaria Majalis is poisonous, but in the correct dilution and potency there is definitely no danger. Very often these sort of things get a wrong interpretation, like the child who drank the seven-day-old water from a vase which contained lily of the valley. This child suffered adverse reactions, i.e. sweating and palpitations, and was generally distressed. It is then that beautiful plants get blamed, because they are used without discretion. But if herbal remedies are taken according to directions and only when they are needed, there are no dangers.

This story disproves statements about natural cures being totally ineffective. One should realise that herbal energy is an energy of vital force which inspires the body to live and often supplies the energy essential to the body when there are problems.

Herbalism aims to treat the patient, not the disease, by directing this vital force and by encouraging and stimulating the body's own defences to produce the desired return to positive health. This is the reason that Convallaria is sometimes mentioned as being good for the senile heart and has produced remarkable results where conventional drugs have failed.

Nettles – Urtica Urens Urens L and Urtica Dioica L

From the beautiful and sweet-smelling, attractive lily of the valley we move on to a plant which is treated as a great enemy in many gardens. Yet it is such a wonderful friend if used not only as a compost for the garden, but also for many diseases and illnesses.

The nettle is virtually indestructable as many gardeners will confirm and we know that on sunny slopes, steep paths and on the rubbish heaps it appears on its own volition. It seems to appear anywhere where it is not wanted. Nettles can be used as garden compost and as a medicinal herb are also valuable.

Not so long ago there was a story in a British newspaper about a lady who was crippled with rheumatism. One day while she was trying to work in the garden, she lost her balance and landed in a bed of stinging nettles. She suffered unwelcome pains and severe itching. However, she noticed the next day that some of the crippling effects in her arms and legs had lessened.

Nettles ease rheumatic pains and are helpful in the cleansing of the blood and beneficial for the composition of the blood. They purify the body and take away inflammations, especially in the urinary passages. I often advise patients to mix some nettles through their salads since they are rich in iron and are beneficial to the digestive system.

A little girl was brought to me with incurable dermatitis. After having tried many things I finally advised the mother to use not only the extract of nettles, but also to put fresh nettles in her soups and salads.

Dr Vogel mentioned in his book *The Nature Doctor* how appropriate it was that nature had given this plant the protection of a stinging exterior. Without it we would probably never have the opportunity to avail ourselves of its healing powers. Animals, with their instinctive knowledge of what is beneficial to them, would not leave any for us were it not for the plant's protective sting. I am sure that it was with this in mind that Dr Vogel created Urticalcin — a calcium remedy which contains the stinging nettle with its abundance of calcium, phosphorous, iron and many other important minerals.

A great friend of mine, a doctor in The Netherlands, and I once had a heated discussion. I told him that Urticalcin was the most effective form of calcium to be absorbed by the body in a patient with calcium deficiency. He did not agree. However, he took the time and trouble to test it and was so pleased with the results that he now uses only Urticalcin for this deficiency problem. In my day-to-day practice it has provided amazing results for people with a calcium deficiency and all the problems resulting from that.

Our great-great-grandfathers used nettles for anaemia, stomach cramps, dropsy and rheumatism. Today nettles are a respected remedy in homoeopathy for urticaria (an allergic skin condition characterised by the appearance of intensely itching weals) and I am sure that our forefathers who might have had rheumatic hands when working in the fields have involuntarily made contact with this plant. Perhaps they have had to discover the hard way what a little injection of the Urtica stinging nettle could do for their condition.

Cornflower – Centaurium Umbellatum

When walking around gardens or herbal gardens I cannot help but stop by this little and attractive blue plant. Respectfully I consider the blessings *Centaurium* may pride itself in. I could not write this chapter and not mention this herb, because having worked with it often I am aware of its medicinal value. In a later book in this series I shall write in more detail about this herb, but I had to include the plant here as it is capable of boosting the general well-being of people.

Centaurium may be used in cases of a weak stomach, sour stomach, indigestion problems, inflammation of mucous membranes of the stomach or for bad appetite. Even with drug-addicts it helps to combat the side-effects. A young girl came to me in despair, not knowing where to turn. She had been on drugs for a long time and had frequently tried to kick the habit, but the nasty side-effects of stomach cramp had always pushed her back. Yet again, Centaurium did not disappoint me. Using this remedy she managed to overcome the side-effects and withdrawal symptoms of which drug users are usually so afraid.

Centaurium Umbellatum is also a help with patients who have a long history of stomach problems and excellent results may be obtained.

Centaurium is a worthy name to remember, as in The Netherlands it has been given the marvellous and apt nickname of *duizend gulden kruid*, which means that the value of this herb was often said to be thousands of guilders. I can honestly say that this herb has surprised even people who had lost their regard for life. It is not purely coincidental that the Romans believed the plant had magical powers, because I have witnessed the results many times. The plant grows easily anywhere, but is often underrated for its capabilities in the treatment of people's ailments.

Feverfew – Tanacetun Partheniun

A while ago I was asked to lecture to a large group of students at a college not far from my practice. I was asked to speak on food and nutrition, but I could not help talking a little about herbal medicine. I tried to instil some respect for nature which God has given us, not only that we may admire the physical beauty of the plants, but also be aware that these same beautiful plants have healing powers.

I picked a few weeds, plants and herbs and took these along with me in a bag. The lecture turned into a horticultural lesson and I was astonished to discover how ignorant these youngsters were about nature. I told them that at that particular time some newspapers were carrying articles about feverfew, because it was said that a doctor's wife had accidentally discovered that this herb had affected her migraines favourably. Since then some research on feverfew has been done and today we use it in herbal medicine for a variety of purposes, amongst others for rheumatic problems.

Feverfew, regarded as a weed in the garden, grows beautifully along the roadside. Its strong smell is reminiscent of medicinal concoctions. *The Family Herbal* written by John Hill MD in 1772 recalls that for the worst headaches, this herb is capable of bringing relief. We may call it the painkiller of all times, because it is as effective as modern painkillers. Luckily feverfew does not display any side-effects and this remedy is therefore prescribed frequently for migraines. The extract of this versatile plant is also used for psychosomatic problems, depression, high spirit problems, pre-menstrual problems and even to dissuade people with suicidal tendencies.

An older lady who had been a patient for many years had been given several different remedies for her complaints, but all to no avail. She had heard from a friend about feverfew but did not know the plant, so I gave her some from my garden. Her arthritic condition was indeed bad, especially in her hands and feet. She chewed three to five leaves per day. These are very bitter, although one does get used to the taste, which is not totally unpleasant. She found that after a few weeks she was able to straighten her hands a bit better. She persevered on this treatment and found it had a tremendous effect on her condition.

When we meet she will always remind me of that episode and repeats to me time and time again: "It was the feverfew that did it". We have to admit again that with all the knowledge we have inherited and gathered on herbal remedies, there are numerous plants which have never been researched. No doubt we will still be able to unravel more secrets through further research, especially as the benefits of feverfew were only discovered by accident.

Periwinkle – Vinca Minor

I could not fail to mention this herbal remedy which is recommended for use in cases of disturbances in the cerebral circulation. It is also valuable in the treatment of lack of concentration, weakness of memory, headache, dizziness, tinnitus (noises in the ears) and difficulties in being able to adapt and communicate, which are generally referred to as behavioural problems. It is also useful for nosebleeds, itching and oozing, rashes, acne, cradlecap and eczema. These ailments are listed in Dr Vogel's *Vademecum*.

The characteristics of periwinkle have been known for some time. In his excellent book *Grandmother's Secrets – Her green guide to health from plants*, Jean Palaiseul writes about health cures which have been derived from plants. This lovely book gives us an extensive guide on herbs, plants and weeds which he researched in his native France. I greatly enjoyed his writing about periwinkle or *Vinca Minor*. He informs us of a letter Mme de Sevigne wrote in 1684 to her daughter: "Lastly my dear, about your health complaints — and the comfort and cures you obtained from your good periwinkle. Very green and very bitter, but very good for your complaints as you already know. It will even cool an inflamed chest."

The particular problems for which Dr Vogel claims periwinkle to be useful in his *Vademecum* are beyond doubt. One has to believe that because of the characteristics and healing properties of *Vinca Minor*, excellent results in all these regions will be obtained. An older friend who was having problems with his memory and concentration claimed to have noticed a marked improvement after a few months of using *Vinca Minor*. Its lilac flowers which are so attractive, have also given relief with unusual problems like ulcers on the tongue, or bleedings which appear spontaneously. Also with skin problems *Vinca Minor* can be of great help. With a persistent eczema, which does not react to specific herbal remedies, we often use *Vinca Minor* successfully.

Lady's mantle – Alchemilla Vulgaris

This chapter on herbs given to us by our Creator to ease human suffering cannot end without my telling you about lady's mantle. It not only grows in grassland and woodlands, but also in mountainous regions. I have often stopped to admire this somewhat kidney-shaped leaf plant when wandering through the Swiss mountains where it grows close to the plant silver lady's mantle. Since Christian times this plant has been greatly admired and has been associated with Mary, the mother of Jesus Christ.

I am sure that the reason it got the name lady's mantle is that the plant has been of great benefit for menstrual disorders and for specific woman's problems. For any female disorders related to menstrual complaints, lady's mantle has been of great benefit. I have also found it helpful particularly for our lady patients who suffer from multiple sclerosis as they tend to be subjected to bladder complaints. It is also useful to people in general who have problems with the connective tissue, hernia problems, weak ligaments or wounds which are difficult to heal. Its healing potential is beyond expectation and again lady's mantle reminds us of the great vital force within each plant to help our own defence system.

In the next chapter we are going to look at what grows *in*

the ground, rather than what grows *above* the ground. In other words we are going to have a look at roots.

3

Roots

Comfrey – Symphytum Officinalis

This herbal root is used nowadays for the treatment of trauma, sport or occupational related injuries, arthritis, distortions, haematomas, phlebitis, swelling of joints, inflamed tendons, tenosynovitis, rheumatic problems, neuritis, tennis elbow, golf elbow, wrinkled skin, intestinal ulcers, gastric and intestinal inflammations of the mucous membranes and so on.

In old herbal treatments the extract of this particular root was used for mending broken bones, to ease bruises, sprains, swellings and backaches. According to an old Elizabethan recipe: boil comfrey root with sugar and liquorice mixed with coltsfoot, mallow and poppy to make an ointment for all these particular problems. Comfrey tea was used for colds and bronchitis. It was very interesting to read that comfrey, which was grown in the gardens of the old monasteries and was used by the monks for the sick and injured was then called "knit-bone". I am often reminded of this in our large osteopathic section of the clinic where we deal with a lot of neck and back problems. Frequently, comfrey, in whatever form, internally as well as externally, has given us reason to admire its healing effects.

Treating particular back and neck problems or injuries and even in the case of fractures, we frequently achieve surprising results when using this particular remedy. When opening the root we see rich and thick liquid oozing from it and with the use of our imagination we can visualise its strong healing powers. If the liquid touches our skin in the course of breaking the root, we can notice that the skin improves. It is an extraordinary characteristic of comfrey — the influence on the skin and wrinkles, crow's feet and ageing skin. No doubt we are dealing with a marvellous remedy, extracted from a root which grows deep down in the earth and without any exterior attraction.

Comfrey is recommended for internal and external use. As I have already mentioned we use this extract often in our osteopathic clinic and are very enthusiastic about the excellent results it has enabled us to achieve.

When I worked in China, I observed that one of the Chinese doctors was very successful with an anti-smoking treatment, but he was very secretive about the acupuncture points he used.

We still come across this professional rivalry a great deal in China. I had asked him several times if he was prepared to share these points with me, but he was adamant he would not divulge the information.

One day during a conversation we touched on the subject of herbs and he asked me if I knew anything about comfrey. As most Chinese doctors are interested in herbal treatments and indeed frequently use them, we discussed some of the qualities peculiar to comfrey. He was interested to find out which way comfrey should be

44

grown. I then suggested some Chinese marketing and perhaps we could trade some information. We struck a deal that I would tell him what I knew about comfrey and he would give me the specific anti-smoking acupuncture points, with which I have been able to help so many people. Since that time we have been in regular correspondence and he has informed me that he has followed my advice regarding the way to grow comfrey and he has also told me about the successes he has achieved with his patients for whom comfrey was prescribed.

The old monks were quite accurate when they called comfrey "knit-bone", because it does knit the tissues together. For thousands of years this remedy has been used to promote healing and recently in homoeopathy it is being used for a wide variety of complaints. I remember an occasion a few years ago which once more made me realise the excellence of this root.

A famous show jumper who was in Scotland for some horse trials, had an unfortunate accident when the horse slipped. She was thrown off, the horse fell on top of her and both rider and horse suffered some rather painful injuries. When she arrived at the hospital, she was told that for some weeks she would not be able to ride and that she would have to take great care even after recovery from her injuries. One of her friends who knew me brought her to me with the horse, which is also well known. First I attended to the rider and prescribed comfrey for both internal and external use for her. Afterwards I examined and treated the horse. Both made a remarkable recovery and when the rider, whose name frequently appears in the national and international press, told me that a week later she wanted to take part in championships to be held in Germany, I gave it some thought before making up my mind. As they had both made such a marvellous recovery I considered that they were well enough to go.

Every day when I pass through my hallway I see the nicely framed saddle cloth which was used for the horse when this combination won the German competition held so shortly after that bad accident.

I could relate many more stories about comfrey and about people I have treated over the years with this remedy. Hundreds of case histories are available to me that could give us an insight into the workings of this herbal root, which gives us such rich medicinal juices. It is not, however, just the root we use, but also the leaves which are used for open wounds like varicose ulcers, for gout, for painful bones and bone fractures.

I like to use comfrey in a combination developed by Dr Vogel. This remedy is called Symphosan and consists of:

Symphytum officinalis	— Comfrey
Hamamelis virg.	— Witchhazel
Hypericum perforatum	— St John's wort
Solidago virg.	— Goldenrod
Sanicula europa	— Sanicle
Sempervivum tectorum	— Houseleek
Arnica montana	— Arnica

Symphosan is a wonderful remedy for the problems I have indicated before and may be used externally for rubbing onto the affected areas, or internally to be taken as drops in some water. It is most unlikely that anyone will be disappointed with the results. Symphosan has been of great help in my practice.

I remember a rather awkward patient who told me that he had a chronic back problem and that there was no way he wanted me to touch his back, either with acupuncture or manipulation, as he had had some bad experiences in the past with several practitioners he had attended. He just wanted my opinion and I could only have a look at his back if I promised that I would not touch it. When I looked at it, my hands were really itching to put a few things in order, but I decided to wait till I had won his confidence. I told him that I would be very careful and that I had years of experience dealing with backs and necks. For the time being I could only prescribe him a good and sensible diet to build up his reserves and I gave him a bottle of Symphosan with instructions for usage.

This man had had chronic problems for more than twenty years and he was in a deplorable condition but, surprisingly, when he came to the end of the second bottle of Symphosan, he entered the consulting-room walking a lot straighter and told me that it had been almost a miracle. He then gave me permission to treat his back and I told him that I would only straighten it out where I considered it necessary. I promised him that I would not take any risks, just as I never would with any patient. Today he is one of the happiest men in the world.

Some time ago a famous singer came to me about problems with her voice, which she felt might be caused by tension in the neck. She was slightly despondent as she suspected that it was affecting her performance. After careful examination I gave her an osteopathic manipulation and advised her to also use Symphosan daily. Nowadays her voice is as good as ever and she is a joy to listen to.

Couch Grass – Triticum Repens

Couch grass is also known as twitch grass, quick grass or squitch. It is considered a great enemy in one's garden. If we watch gardeners desperately trying to get rid of the couch grass in their gardens, we soon realise that they will never succeed in doing so unless they manage to remove the roots. It is the root in particular that I want to tell you about.

Although these roots are such a pest in our gardens,

they can also be an ally. In olden days the juices from the couch grass roots were used for all kinds of problems ranging from gout and rheumatism, to acne and other skin conditions. Today couch grass has very much gone out of fashion as once it was used to rub on the skin to improve conditions and heal inflammations. However, even with present-day problems it may be used successfully and I would like to mention *Lupus Erythematosus* which today seems to be getting more and more publicity.

Someone from the Midlands phoned me about a girl who had an unidentified problem and asked me to examine this girl and advise her. When I saw her I knew that this could be a case of *Lupus Erythematosus* and I asked her doctor to perform certain hospital tests to find out if this diagnosis was correct. Those tests were performed and the diagnosis was confirmed. One of the opinions was that this could have been caused by radiation, which of course could not be proven. When I asked what action had been decided upon I was informed that the only way to treat her conventionally was with cortisone. I examined the girl again and contacted an old doctor friend. Much to my surprise he advised me to treat her with remedies like comfrey and Petasites, but added that she should be instructed to drink daily two half glasses of the juice of the roots of couch grass.

As she had reached an advanced stage of this illness, her doctor did not object, but of course it was difficult to gather sufficient couch grass roots. Fortunately everyone co-operated and as other orthodox remedies failed, we started this treatment. My old doctor friend warned me however that she might have to go through a heavy crisis and this is exactly what happened. One evening while attending a medical conference in London, I was informed by telephone that she had a temperature of nearly 104°F and that she had contracted pneumonia. However, after battling through the night she came through the crisis and after a few weeks it was hard to recognise her as the same person.

She recovered very well and a few years later when I saw her, she told me that she had decided to study medicine. I was very grateful and realised once again how much nature has to offer. What is discarded in our gardens is not necessarily useless. Although the medical properties of couch grass have largely been forgotten, nowadays there are indeed many complaints to which this root is applicable.

Two other roots come to mind and have been greatly used in my practice. Neither of them originate from Europe. The first is a root which has recently come into the limelight in western countries.

Devil's Claw – Harpagophytum

The reason for the name devil's claw is that the seeds of this particular plant are finger-like growths which are protected by thorns and have a strange appearance. However devil's claw, which has today become well known, has been used for therapeutic treatments by the natives of Namibia for centuries. In many magazines on nature cures, this root is often recommended for the cleansing of the kidneys.

The attraction of the root is that it does not contain any toxic substances. The result is that it is suitable for all-round cleansing of the organs and it has a good diuretic influence. It is also recommended for use in cases of angina pectoris and arteriosclerosis. In many reports on herbal medicine in Britain today we find wonderful testimonies from patients with long-established rheumatism or arthritis histories who have experienced great relief from this root-based treatment.

Dr Vogel states in one of his articles that the root of this plant is the most favourable remedy with people all over the world. It gives the body a thorough cleansing and acts as a preventive measure against any possible undesirable illness. Lately I have found it most helpful in cases of patients suffering with allergies. Together with a few complementary remedies it is also known to help in cases of neuritis (inflammation of the nerves), diabetes, urticaria (hives), thrombosis and cardio-vascular disease.

For the first time in history a faculty of the University of Utrecht in The Netherlands held a very interesting symposium in 1985 to discover the therapeutic value of plant products. The interaction and development of plant products are of great importance and I am pleased to see the interest in a more multi-directional approach.

Temoe Lawak – Curcuma Xanthorrhiza

Temoe Lawak has been used for medicinal purposes for centuries. The reason lies in its ability to purify the blood by the removal of bile. Few other plants have been observed to possess this action. Temoe Lawak is the Malayan name for plants belonging to the family of Zingiberaceae. An extract is obtained from the roots and tubers. The plants are chiefly found in tropical regions. They range in height between 50 and 200 cms and have fleshy, creeping, branched underground rhizomes with many tuberous roots.

The leaves of the plant are arranged in two slanting rows. The upper surface is green with a reddish-brown area in the centre. Numerous small flowers are carried on stout stalks. The plant with which we are concerned is *Curcuma Xanthorrhiza*, one of the genus Curcuma. The group of plants described is characterised by the presence of essential oils. The Curcuma plants also contain a mixture of yellow pigments known as curcumins. The oils and pigments are the most important elements in Temoe Lawak.

Temoe Lawak has been used successfully for hundreds of years. It was widely employed in the treatment of yellow jaundice, partly because of its yellow colour (which is imparted by the curcumins), but partly because of the resemblance between the plant rhizomes and the gallbladder. Temoe Lawak is an excellent example of a medicine whose use is based on physical properties, in this case the twin properties of colour and shape.

The use of plants of the genus Curcumus dates from ancient times. Curcuma are referred to in the Old Testament and Marco Polo was familiar with them. In the eighteenth century they were included in a number of pharmaceutical reference books. Around 1900, the Dutch introduced *Curcuma Xanthorrhiza* to the European market under the name Temoe Lawak.

From ancient times, the Curcuma have been used as dyes, spices and medicines, particularly in the countries of origin. As dyes, they are widely used for colouring silk and leather, but also foodstuffs such as cheese and mustard. In the realm of spices, they are found among others in curry powder, turmeric, coriander, cinnamon and ginger. As a medicinal root, Curcuma is among the best-selling items in the Indonesian spice merchant's stock. On the island of Java, it is to be found in practically every compound remedy.

Temoe Lawak is a preparation with both cholekinetic (gallbladder-evacuating) and choleretic (bile-forming) properties. The yellow pigments are primarily responsible for the cholekinetic action, and the essential oil for the stimulation of bile formation.

Many of the foods which we eat are too high in cholesterol. It is vital to break down these fatty acids. The essential oil in Temoe Lawak assists in dissolving cholesterol. It also has disinfectant properties. Temoe Lawak therefore has a beneficial action, particularly in cases of inflammation of the bile ducts and gallstones.

It has recently been discovered that the Curcuma possess anti-microbial properties. By slowing the rate of growth of certain bacteria, they arrest inflammation of tissues. Some of these bacteria were suspected of playing a part in the incidence of cancer of the intestines. The possibility of a connection was thoroughly investigated by The Netherlands Institute for Applied Physical Research (TNO). The results of their laboratory research were such as to justify further study.

Since 1947 Temoe Lawak has been produced in tablet form. This is much more practical and also meets objections on the part of some users concerning the taste. Temoe Lawak has long been a household word in South-east Asia. The tea made from rhizomes of the Curcuma was effective against yellow jaundice and for dispersing gallstones. It subsequently transpired that Temoe Lawak could play a major part in regulating the entire biliary metabolism. Temoe Lawak also helps to arrest inflammation. The ability of Temoe Lawak to regulate the biliary metabolism has led to the idea that it could also be used to suppress, or even prevent, attacks of migraine.

4

Seeds

WHEN WE think about seeds we have to consider the problems concerning saturated fatty acids. Unrefined oils contain highly unsaturated fatty acids and we should bear in mind that research has shown how vital it is that our dietary habits be changed. The use of olive-oil, sunflowerseed-oil, soya-oil, oil from nuts such as walnuts, pine kernels and even apricot kernels, is much more preferable to using refined oils. Excellent supplies of unsaturated fatty acids are available even in the smaller seeds like sesame seeds and we should make an effort to realise how important this is for our health.

I am always surprised to find the part seeds play in the daily diet of primitive peoples and I enjoy seeing the good health that results from the chewing of these seeds, even the simplest seeds such as the pip from apple, grapefruit or lemon. Although this should not be done indiscriminately, it certainly will be rewarding as an investment in our health.

I personally like using and working with linseeds but they should be ground well before use. They may also be chewed, but do make sure that they are fresh. Mixed with several other products such as honey or savoury herbs they have beneficial effects. Linseeds or flaxseeds stimulate a good bowel movement and hundreds of patients with a constipation problem have experienced great relief from the use of Dr Vogel's remedy Linoforce.

Linum usitatissium is one of the oldest cultivated plants in existence, grown throughout the world. It contains 3-6% acidy mucilage which is located in the skin of the seed shell. When fully ripened, the seeds have the most mucilage, which is especially important for a laxative effect. Furthermore, flaxseed contains approximately 25% protein, 30-40% fatty oil, sugar, sterine and cyanogenic glycoside (Linamarin).

There is no need to be concerned about poisoning, since the linamarase splits to a slight degree only, due to the pH of the stomach. Even in the case of upset acidity conditions, the speed of elimination of the hydro-cyanide acid is substantially greater than the separation process, which extends over a period of several hours. The effectiveness of the flaxseed lies, on the one hand, in its ability to expand (expansion of the mucilage in the seed shell epidermis) whereby, thanks to the increase in volume, the peristaltic reflexes are stimulated. On the other hand the mucilage has an enveloping effect, reducing irritation and blocking reabsorption.

It forms a protective layer over the mucous membrane. Painful and inflammatory processes are influenced indirectly in a favourable manner by this soothing and inflammation-blocking effect. This also prevents the anthraquinone-glycoside contained in Linoforce from excessively irritating the muscular structure of the bowel. At the same time a deodorising characteristic, i.e. a property that blocks the growth of a decaying agent in the bowel, can be ascribed to flaxseed (possibly due to the low amounts of hydro-cyanide being released).

Another seed which is of great importance is the sunflower seed. These seeds today do not receive the recognition they warrant. We have noticed that sunflower seeds in the treatment of multiple sclerosis patients are very beneficial. This is not only a tasty seed, it contains highly unsaturated oils and is very rich in vitamins and minerals, amongst others Vitamins A and B and iron, calcium and smaller amounts of other minerals.

The sunflower seeds are helpful in educating children to develop healthy dietary habits. Mixed with fruits and nuts they can be offered to children as a tasty snack, which will give them a healthy supply of vitamins and minerals. Sunflower seeds are also used in the manufacture of sunflower-oil and as the name would suggest sunflower-oil margarine. These products are recommended before products containing saturated fatty acids.

If we think of sunflower seeds, we automatically think of poppy seeds. Many different kinds of bread available today have poppy seeds on top, but it is not enough to eat just a few poppy seeds used for the decoration of our bread. Poppy seeds are eaten in certain countries on specific feast days and they should be considered an easy and pleasant way to increase our vitamin and mineral intake. Poppy seeds would make an ideal substitute in cases of mineral or vitamin deficiencies and it is a good idea that from time to time poppy seeds are eaten in combination with other foods. A delicious spread may be prepared from poppy seeds which are a nice complement to wholemeal bread.

Did you know that the sesame seed contains very little oil? How lovely these seeds are in the sesame/honey bars which we can buy in the health food shop, but are you aware that these little seeds contain an abundance of minerals such as iron, potassium, calcium and vitamins? The highly unsaturated acid of the sesame seeds is easily assimilated in our cells and tissues and forms a very nutritious food substance. Not only are sesame seeds tasty, they are also a very good remedy in combating constipation, eczema and other defensive problems of the body. Dr Vogel writes in his book *The Nature Doctor* that sesame seeds are also good for patients afflicted with liver and gallbladder problems.

Again it is very important that these seeds are chewed well. If one is in possession of an electric food processor or a liquidiser, a lovely creamy mixture can be produced by blending together sesame seeds, figs, apples, oranges, rosehips and sunflower seeds. It really makes a delicious and very rich, healthy mixture.

From the rich supply of seeds I would like to mention one, which is of considerable value in the treatment of problems typical of this day and age. I am referring to the freshly extracted oil from the seeds of the evening-primrose. This is beneficial to people suffering from multiple sclerosis, incidences of which are unfortunately increasing. Skin problems, eczema, menopausal complaints, post-operative complications, slow-healing wounds and scars are also aided by oil of evening-primrose. In fact, the oil of evening-primrose has been a wonderful discovery. Frequently, where other remedies have failed to bring improvement with various problems, the oil of evening-primrose has done so with tremendous effect.

I was consulted by a lady who underwent a surgical operation four years ago. Since then she has suffered some bad pains as a result of scar tissue damage. The surgeon who operated tried to help her in every way, but without success. I attempted to help her with acupuncture, which unfortunately only gave her temporary relief. Then I decided in addition to put her on a high dosage of oil of evening-primrose capsules. During a subsequent visit she informed me that for the first time in over four years she was now totally without pain.

In my earlier book on multiple sclerosis I have given plenty of evidence of the capabilities of the oil of evening-primrose. These little seeds of the evening-primrose remind me of a phrase from an old poem which says:

Life unseen,
by moonlight shades in valleys green
lovely flower will live unseen.

Although very small, these seeds have become of great value.

Let us not forget that the very largest tree we might ever see in our life started as a result of the tremendous vital force which is present in every little seed and which can grow to aid and protect life. If we look at nature from this angle, it is almost impossible to comprehend.

During question time after a lecture I held in South Africa for a large medical gathering, a gentleman stood up and asked me for my opinion and advice on the use of seeds and herbs which were given to us in the Bible. He felt that we had ignored our original diet of fruits and seeds which have been made available to us. He also said that the Creator of all mankind commanded that we eat the plants of the field.

There was a considerable change in the original diet after the Flood but certainly I agreed with this gentleman that seeds contain the vital source of energy, which is of the utmost importance to our health. I reminded him of seeds like the coriander seed, which had been compared to manna, which God fed his people in the wilderness on their way to the promised land. Coriander seed, which is so rich in vitamins and minerals, is also a marvellous appetiser and a very good remedy for the stomach. In olden days it was also used for rheumatism, painful joints and caries (decays of bones or teeth).

In my reply to the gentleman who had asked my opinion

and advice I also mentioned mustard seed. Are we familiar with the wonderful properties of the mustard seed?

An old lady, whose only income was her old-age pension, came to see me about her rheumatic and arthritic problems. I advised her to take the juice of a raw potato, about which I will write more in a later chapter dealing with vegetables, and ten or twelve mustard seeds every morning. It was wonderful to see that after about six weeks her crippled hands started to straighten themselves slightly and she told me that since taking the mustard seeds and potato juice her pain had become less severe.

Mustard seeds are not only helpful with rheumatic problems, but can also be useful as a digestive aid. They stimulate the flow of the gastric juices. People who suffer from rheumatic or lumbago pains should take a hot bath to which some mustard seeds have been added. This they will find extremely relaxing and soothing. Some lady patients have experienced relief from vaginal problems with the help of a mustard bath. A poultice of powdered mustard seeds is advised for certain skin problems, but do take care not to make the poultice too strong or it might burn the skin.

Again we see that the very small mustard seed, black as well as white, deserves its place in the kingdom of seeds and should not be underrated.

5

Berries and Currants

IF WE TAKE a walk through nature's kingdom we cannot fail to notice the many berries and currants which grow, but if only we realised how rich in vitamins these are we would perhaps use them more often in our daily diet. They not only contain a considerable amount of Vitamin C, but also an enormous variety of minerals and trace elements, for which there is a great need in our daily diets.

Not only are the well-known raspberries, strawberries, redcurrants and cranberries excellent sources of vitamins, experience has shown that these berries are also very good for the liver, pancreatic disturbances, lymphatic conditions and allergic conditions, where the use of berries can be a bonus.

The most popular of all berries is the strawberry. However, we have to be careful with the strawberry as some people are allergic to it and it can affect the kidneys. It all depends on the way in which strawberries are grown and whether the right manure or compost is used, as cultivated strawberries may sometimes cause a rash. In this respect my old gardener has found a few ways of growing strawberries to which there will be little or no danger of an allergic reaction. If grown his way and if allergic reactions still appear with these cultivated strawberries, then one has to try the wild ones, because there is even less danger of these being harmful.

Strawberry – Fragaria vesca

Strawberries are one of the tastiest berries we can find. They have a high iron content and are often advised for use by people who are anaemic. Not only are they rich in vitamins and iron, they may also be used externally for toning up the skin and if there is no allergic reaction, this is a very good method of improving the complexion. It is not only the fruits of the strawberry plants that are used, even the leaves may be used for the purpose of easing the process of giving birth and tea brewed from the roots of the strawberry may be used for diarrhoea, cystitis and other inflammatory conditions.

Strawberries are greatly loved in Britain. Certainly in Scotland most monasteries in the olden days had great strawberry patches and all the estate gardens today have significant strawberry fields within their walls. I don't think that there are many small domestic gardens which do not have a bed of strawberries in the areas of Lanarkshire, Ayrshire and East Lothian where strawberries are grown in great volume.

Strawberry cultivation however will only be successful if the soil has been properly prepared. The picking of strawberries also needs care. I remember one of my older gardeners who had a patch for strawberries prepared with artificial manure and another patch with organic manure. When the strawberries were ripe, he gave me two bowls with strawberries and asked me if I could notice the difference between the contents of each bowl. I could not fail to immediately notice a difference in the smell, but the difference in taste later was beyond words. The ones he had grown the old-fashioned way in good organic manure were more tasty with a superior smell and could be eaten, I am sure, without any allergic effects.

My gardener taught me that before starting to dig manure into the ground, a two-foot trench should be dug and the soil should be barrelled to the far end of the ground to fill in the trench at the finish of the spadework. As much manure should be dug into the trenches as they will hold and the entire patch should be worked over like this. When the whole patch is well prepared with the manure mixed with some liquid extracted from nettles, the young plants are to be put in. Plant these along either side of a string, stretched along the ground. This should be done in autumn. When spring comes and the plants start to show through there will be no plants to equal them for growth. They will be thick and bushy, but there should not be a single flower on them. After all it is said that young plants should not be allowed to flower during the first year. The following years they will be absolutely laden with fruit and the size of the strawberries will be fantastic. In this particular instance the substantial manure or compost spreading will pay off.

There are lots of ways to grow strawberries. One way which is used by some people is to train the runners between the rows of plants and when they want to renew the beds and manure, they dig in the old plants which of course saves them a lot of work. Another method is to grow the strawberries on a raised bed without planting them in rows and just let them grow naturally. Give them a handful of general fertiliser in the spring. There is no doubt, however, that even if this fertiliser is satisfactory to the plant, if it is a chemical fertiliser it will never produce quite the same quality berries as when an organic fertiliser is used. Without substantial feeding, and I mean natural feeding, one can never expect a first-class quality berry. If no natural feeding is used, strawberries are more likely to cause allergic reactions.

If the strawberry fields are so big that the manure cannot be dug in by hand, then obviously a plough is the answer, as has been done for years by the British farmers who know only too well the technique involved. Strawberries do however thrive on a little bit of tidiness and if we pay them the attention they warrant, we can expect a very good crop.

Strawberries can also be laid down for a number of years and it is important to keep them as free from weeds as possible. I hate to see gardeners who are working their strawberry patches with a cigarette dangling from their lips. Not to speak of the cigarette-ends which will end up in the soil. It is very important to keep any untidiness and rubbish away and to treat strawberries with great care.

There are many varieties of strawberry. The old well-known ones are the Scarlet Queen, which is a fine open plant, the Royal Sovereign and the King George. There are many others and especially some which stand up well to the winter climate, like the Huxley Giant or the Auchencruive Climax. Personally I like the alpine strawberries which are small, wild and a little sweet, but a very good strawberry which is also well accepted by people who show an allergic tendency to strawberries.

My dear old gardener tells me that since he started his gardening career many years ago he has seen many varieties of strawberries. Some kinds have disappeared altogether, especially the climbing varieties which grow up walls. He tells me that very often the birds were his greatest rivals, but as a keen ornithologist he let them get away with it. At one time he realised he was losing most of his strawberries and would find them in heaps among the rows, for which he blamed mice or rats. However, one morning he found the culprit red-handed and discovered that it was a red squirrel storing them away for future use.

I started this chapter with strawberries because of their traditional use and popularity and I will now turn to other berries.

Barberry – *Berberis vulgaris*

If we wander through the valleys we are bound to come across the barberry. Again this berry possesses healing powers and is rich in Vitamin C. Its medicinal properties may be used advantageously in cases of bleeding gums and mouth ulcers. It is a natural follow-up to continue from the barberry to another berry with medicinal value.

Blackberry – *Rubus fruticosus*

Who does not know the blackberry which is still better known in Scotland as the bramble? It is a wonderful gift of God's creation. This native and natural inhabitant of our woodlands, hedgerows and odd corners, grows anywhere and everywhere. Many of us will remember being taken for Sunday outings during the late summer armed with containers or buckets to pick blackberries with which our mothers would later make bramble jelly or jam.

Blackberries are beneficial and a delicious treat for children as well as adults. Not only is blackberry jam, syrup, jelly or pie enjoyed by almost everyone, it is also of medicinal help to the mucous membranes of the throat, irritation of the vocal chords and even for diarrhoea. I remember well when as a child we had a stomach complaint or diarrhoea, that my mother would immediately give us some brown rice with bramble jelly or juice.

TRADITIONAL HOME AND HERBAL REMEDIES

Blackcurrant – Ribes nigrum

The blackcurrant is domestically grown in many British gardens and also extremely popular. The blackcurrant drink or sweet is a popular remedy for a cold or flu and it is also widely used for home wine-making.

Redcurrant – Ribes rubrum

The redcurrant together with the blackcurrant is used to make our delicious redcurrant jelly, which is often domestically produced and enjoyed by many families. Rightly, this may also be classed as a medicinal currant as it is rich in vitamins and the juice of the redcurrant is an excellent mouthwash.

Elderberry – Sambucus nigra

The elderberry was described by Father Kneipp as a faithful family friend. It may be used for medicinal purposes and is one of the most popular berries for the wine-making enthusiasts. Again this berry contains lots of vitamins and minerals and is also suitable for jam-making.

The elderberry wine is said to have twelve characteristics:
1 It is good for indigestion;
2 It stimulates a good, clear urine flow;
3 It makes a white nose nice and red;
4 It gives a good fragrance;
5 It stimulates natural childbirth;
6 It is good for the blood;
7 It produces a nice, natural heat;
8 It gives good hope;
9 It makes people courageous;

10 It helps people forget sadness and misery;

11 It makes people less mean;

12 It makes old men and women young again.

Because of these twelve characteristics the elderberry is largely used in Britain for wine and jam-making and unfortunately not very often for its medicinal properties.

Raspberry – *Rubus idoeus*

The wild raspberry, or Mount Ida bramble, has been hunted for many years and is much sought after, especially in Scotland. The wild raspberry grows like the blackberry and it is also used for jam-making. The greatest care must be taken however when gathering wild raspberries as they attract wasps who build their nests in the bushes.

The raspberry is a delicious berry and many farms, particularly in Perthshire where a lot of raspberries are grown, employ a good deal of occasional labour during the summer months. It is nice to see that people can go and pick their own raspberries on these farms as in this way we can all share the healthy substances contained in these berries.

In old books on herbal medicine raspberries were often recommended for people with nervous dispositions or those suffering from insomnia. Raspberry tea is good for menstrual problems and it also alleviates the pains of childbirth. Mixed with other berries it makes a delicious drink, which will provide a good and healthy sleep. Raspberries also make a refreshing summer dessert when mixed with redcurrants.

Rowanberry – *Sorbus aucuparia*

Now I turn to a more accepted medicinal berry, namely the rowanberry. It is in autumn that the rowantree produces her beautiful red berries. I sometimes feel sorry for people who have throat problems or suffer from hoarseness, as the rowanberry would clear this up in no time.

Unfortunately it is generally considered to be a poisonous berry. Granted, if one eats the rowanberry indiscriminately, it may be detrimental to one's health. It may however be used medicinally with great success. How grateful an old gentleman patient was after I had advised him to chew some rowanberries every day, when he was able to tell me that the hoarseness from which he had suffered for years had completely disappeared.

The rowanberry, together with the rosehip and the barberry, makes a pleasant and healthy dessert that is an ideal combination when suffering throat problems.

Dr Vogel and I once took a large group of medical students on a nature ramble. Dr Vogel picked some rowanberries and started eating them, explaining to the students that his voice would benefit. These students were watching him in horror, convinced of the fact that Dr Vogel was poisoning himself. He remarked however that the birds who enjoy the taste of rowanberries do not die and they will do human beings no harm if they are used with common sense. It will, in fact, be to their advantage.

Juniperberry – Juniperus communis

The juniperberry has been popular through the ages and was grown in the old monasteries for many, many years. Juniperberries were also used in wines in the olden days. The wine is sure to have been a great attraction to our forefathers as the old herbalists claimed that the juniperberry would give us longevity. The berries have a bitter-sweet constituent, but are very good for rheumatism, nephritis (kidney disease), asthma, bladder problems and to keep one's mind fresh and young. This last quality was again a reason why the juniperberry used to be so popular.

This unusual tasting berry has earned great praise from the old herbalists who claimed that it stimulated the appetite, cleansed the stomach and is of benefit to the glands.

Juniper-oil, which is derived from the berries, penetrates the skin and is beneficial when used in cases of bone/joint problems and if added to the bath-water or to a steam-bath it is very useful for bronchial infections.

Hawthorn – Crataegus oxyecantha

Lastly in this chapter on berries and currants I would like to mention the benefits which have been enjoyed over the centuries from the hawthorn berry. In a fresh herb preparation this berry deals with complaints of a nervous heart, it strengthens cardiac activity and tones and regulates an over-excited or stimulated heart. It always pleases me to hear the many stories regarding the hawthorn. When we look at the berries hanging in bunches from the thorny bushes along the roadside, we perhaps do not realise of what assistance the hawthorn has been over the ages for many people suffering from the abovementioned complaints.

Dr Vogel developed Crataegisan, a most harmless and reliable remedy, which may be taken together with arnica or in combination with other remedies. As such it has been a blessing for people who suffer from heart palpitations and anxiety.

Even in Biblical days we read about the hawthorn, but still today in medical science the hawthorn is recognised as valuable in many serious problems. I remember a lady who was told by her doctors to live a very quiet life as she had a weak heart and there was not much they could do for her. Among other things there were signs of high blood pressure, hardening of the arteries and angina pectoris.

I remember her well as she was one of the earlier patients I treated in Britain and because of her great spirit and attitude to life I became very fond of her. Her blood pressure was very irregular and after trying several remedies, I decided to put her on a low dosage of Crataegisan. She responded wonderfully and much to everyone's surprise was able to attend her daughter's wedding. She continued to use Crataegisan and has learned to respect it through her own experience. It has been a blessing to her.

An Irish lady who attended my clinic just recently told me that she had got a new lease of life since I advised her to use hawthorn regularly and that she felt unable to express her gratitude. In the olden days herbalists described the qualities of the hawthorn: "It forms a good extra belt round the heart for those who need it"

Of all the wonderful berries which appear in nature, we have only discussed a few, but we again realise that we should be thankful to nature for the medicinal value of these berries. I look at people who once sat in my consulting-room with heart problems and who were forced to change their pace of life. All along a simple remedy like Crataegus was supplied by nature to improve their condition, if only we had not strayed so far from the natural way.

6

Vegetables

HIPPOCRATES said it so well: "Let your food be medicine, and your medicine, food!" This is very much the case with vegetables and although we look on vegetables as a daily food, it is not so likely that we look on them as a medicine. How true this is if we realise that vegetables are really purpose-grown herbs.

Our cultivated vegetables originally were wild plants and though today they are both specialised and cultivated, they should still be considered as a food which also can be a medicine. In this respect I often advise patients to examine wild vegetables. These wild vegetables, as we call them, are of particular interest to me in this chapter, as they have often been used for their medicinal properties. Out of the enormous variety of everyday vegetables we find on our table, and of all the lesser used wild vegetables, I can only select a few to discuss here. Of necessity I will restrict myself to those vegetables which I have been able to use as part of my patients' treatment.

People who live in the jungle need a lot more resilience for their way of life, and they exist on wild vegetables. We, as supposedly cultured people, could learn a lesson from them as in our day and age the quality of our vegetables has deteriorated. It is not so much the quantity of vegetables we eat, but the quality which is important.

The health value of vegetables today depends completely on the quality of the soil in which they are grown. Luckily organic farming is becoming more popular today and soil cultivated with the right compost is receiving more attention. In our own nursery I have followed the growing of our vegetables with great interest. We use organic compost and the quality of the resulting vegetable is excellent. It is also interesting to note that very often not only the quality but also the quantity of the vegetable is better when the right organic compost is used. It is a proven fact that vegetables grown with organic compost contain greater amounts of vitamins, minerals and trace elements, than is the case when treated with artificial fertiliser.

I look at the results which come back from the agricultural college where tests are done on the produce we grow. I am delighted with these results, but it is also the smell and taste of our home-grown produce which pleases me. Garden produce grown the old-fashioned or bio-dynamic way cannot be beaten.

Dr Vogel once showed me two cherry trees, one of which was over 50 years old, laden with fruit, bearing a good-quality cherry, very tasty and attractive. The cherries might not have been the most beautiful I had ever seen, but the taste was absolutely magnificent. The other tree was much younger, the leaves were greener and the cherries looked beautiful, but the taste of the cherry was inferior to that of the first tree. This second tree had been fed artificial fertiliser. Dr Vogel wanted to show me the difference between the size of the cherry produced and the quality of the taste. The leaves were greener and the younger tree should have had more fruit than the older tree. This confirms my feeling that today not enough thought is given to the health and well-being of people, or rather that it is channelled in the wrong direction.

Organic gardening is something we desperately need today to strengthen our immune systems with plentiful supplies of vitamins, minerals and trace elements. So often garden produce is spoilt by all this artificial fertilising and the use of pesticides and insecticides, which are so harmful to our health. For goodness sake, let us be careful with the treatment of the vegetable, one of our main sources of food. If we treat it with respect and value it, it will serve us well.

I recently read a book called *The Secret Life of Plants*, written by Peter Tomkins and Christopher Birds. I enjoyed the book and several items mentioned therein were of use to me in underlining what I am trying to put over here. I read that a chemist, Marcel Vogel, researched if, and how, man is linked with plant life. He stated in one of his lectures: "Man can and does communicate with plant life. Plants are living objects, sensitively rooted in space. They may be blind, deaf and dumb in the human sense, but there is no doubt that they are extremely sensitive instruments for measuring Man's emotions. They radiate energy forces which are beneficial to man. They feed into their own force fields, which in turn feeds energy back to the plant."

Considering this we realise that the life force of our vegetables has to be nurtured, as Marcel Vogel stated in his lecture. We become aware of this if we look at a particular wild vegetable which in my view has a marvellous aroma — the leek. Culzean Castle is one of the oldest estates in Scotland, which once had a beautiful herb garden full of interesting plant life. Whenever I visit these gardens I can smell immediately the aromatic, almost penetrating, tang of wild garlic and wild leeks.

TRADITIONAL HOME AND HERBAL REMEDIES

The wild leek can be of such medicinal influence for a diabetic patient and its extract is used by diabetics over and over again with great results. I remember a good friend of the family who contracted a low degree of diabetes, but did not as yet need insulin. He came to me to ask if there was anything he could do to get his condition under control. I gave him some dietary information and recommended that he use daily some wild leeks and Molkosan (which I will discuss in a later chapter dealing with seasoning). He thrived on this course of action.

And what about the ever-increasing threat of the hated shingles nowadays? Many patients have experienced what it is to suffer from the dreadful pain of shingles. The relief obtained by dabbing the affected areas with wild leek extract has to be experienced to be believed. An older lady came to me recently and thanked me from the bottom of her heart. When she had consulted me previously about her shingles I had given her some homoeopathic remedies and also had advised her to dab the affected areas with the extract from the wild leek. Thankfully she had experienced great relief. Cultivated leeks may also be used to alleviate the effects of this problem.

Wild as well as cultivated leeks are beneficial in cases of high blood pressure and the strength, the power and the vital force which Marcel Vogel describes so beautifully as the secret life in the plant, is there for all to witness.

I am occasionally asked why I am so fond of watercress, as I frequently advise large quantities of this to be included in diets, especially for weight reduction. I add watercress to the daily diet, not only because of its vitamin, mineral and trace element value, but because it is so rich in iodine. The thyroid and other endocrine glands flourish on iodine and it is of benefit to people who battle with weight problems.

Watercress is an ideal way to garnish our food attractively with its pleasant aroma, good taste and looks.

Add to this the bonus of being conducive to good health. Who could turn down a watercress sandwich? A combination of watercress and other vegetables together with some Herbamare seasoning salt, makes a delicious snack, which can be eaten by overweight people without fear, as watercress influences the function of the thyroid.

A nice and light side-salad alongside our cooked vegetables could contain for example watercress, parsley and celery, mixed with some herbs like thyme, oregano or nasturtium. Add a little mint and we have an extremely healthy and tasteful dish.

Now we turn to carrots, which are excellent for our gallbladder and liver. In some parts of the world carrots are always on the menu, because they make such a good balance for the metabolic system. They are ideal for children because of their Vitamin A content and fortunately most children enjoy the taste of them. Carrots can also serve as a preventive measure to rheumatism and arthritis and are also helpful when treating those suffering from impetigo (a contagious skin disease). One of the most unpleasant problems — Meniere's syndrome (a disease of the inner-ear characterised by recurrent attacks of deafness, tinnitus, vertigo, nausea and vomiting) can also be eased by this dietary aid.

Carrots, together with onions and leeks, are of benefit to those who suffer from problems with worms and threadworms. Throughout Britain the carrot has always been grown easily and well and even "spare-time" gardeners manage to produce some wonderful crops. Although it is said that the carrot cannot be transplanted, this is not true as it can actually be transplanted very well. It is a vegetable which should not be omitted when planning the contents of one's vegetable garden, as it has been shown to be of such great value.

Now let us look at the cabbage. No matter where one

went in the past, no matter which estate garden, nursery or small-holding, cabbages were to be found growing everywhere. My gardener tells me that if some systematic thinking were to be done before planting, cabbages could be grown to cover our needs over the entire year. For example, it never does any good planting a summer variety and expecting it to be ready for use in March or April of the following Spring. Some varieties do however have a dual purpose.

Savoury cabbages were also once widely grown and could be seen thriving in gamekeepers' gardens as well as in the big estate gardens. Cabbages were planted in the fields by hand and this operation was undertaken with care and attention by a considerable number of workers. They were seldom watered into the ground, but would lie limp for a few days after which they began to recover. Nowadays we have developed labour-saving methods and cabbages are planted by drills, but the resulting cabbages will be unable to match the quality of those planted by hand.

Cabbage will improve and cure conditions such as arthritis, stomach and metabolic problems. It is rich in calcium and therefore advantageous to correcting our inherent deficiencies. As I like to eat cabbage in its own juices there is no problem with indigestion, which is a possibility with boiled cabbage.

When I think about cabbage, sauerkraut comes to mind. This is white cabbage put through a fermenting process. It is not only a delicious but also an extremely healthy vegetable. Sauerkraut, which is easily prepared, often appears on the menu in hospitals in The Netherlands once or twice a week. Apart from the lemon, sauerkraut is the best anti-scorbutic remedy as Dr Vogel mentions in *The Nature Doctor*, and as we all learned at school in our history lessons, this method was used by James Cook to enable him to sail the farthest seas without any of his men falling victim to scurvy.

As it is easily digested, a spoonful of sauerkraut every day can be of benefit to problems of the mucous membranes, teeth or even with swollen ankles or general weaknesses. Sauerkraut may be used in a poultice for stomach aches or to relieve any feelings of cramp.

With swellings or bruises the response to a cabbage-leaf poultice is remarkable. Fresh cabbage-leaf compresses will aid headaches and sinus trouble. In our osteopathic clinic I treat many swollen ankles and osteo-arthritic or rheumatoid-arthritic knees. I have often been laughed at when I advise patients to place, on alternate nights, a kaolin or a cabbage-leaf poultice on the affected spot. This old-fashioned remedy is simple and very effective. On the first evening before going to bed bandage on the affected area a kaolin poultice and leave on all night. The following evening place fresh cabbage leaves on the area and when bandaged this should also be left till the next morning. The results will not disappoint the user.

A little while ago one of the local doctors stopped me in the street with a big smile on his face. He mentioned the matron of a local nursing home whom I had advised to use these poultices on her knee and said with a bit of a sneer: "I know that you sometimes use the most strange remedies, but at least you are intelligent and have done a lot of studying and training. How in the world can you then believe that you can treat the osteo-arthritic knees of the matron with a cabbage leaf?" I had a little chuckle, but told him that often the old remedies were based on long experience. Knowledge of these natural powers has been handed down for generations and because these methods have been discarded for so long, that does not mean they don't function any more. Dr Vogel states that the healing powers which can bring such relief can be affected by supplying curative elements to the tissues and by eliminating toxics and other harmful substances from these tissues.

Even the Greeks wrote about the medicinal powers of the cabbage leaf and in those days it was known as an important herbal medicine. In old folk medicine the use of cabbage leaves went from generation to generation. Back in 1881 the French doctor Blanc wrote a book about some of his experiences using the cabbage leaf for therapeutic purpose. Dr Blanc who was teaching at a faculty in Paris and also working as a doctor in a hospice at Trone, France, stated: "The cabbage leaf is the doctor of the poor". He listed many options in his book about the capabilities of the cabbage leaf. The Romans were also known to use the cabbage as a universal remedy and it was used to cure many ailments.

The English doctor Head, in the last century, came to the conclusion that segments in the body which were in contact with the spine, can be influenced quite easily through the skin. This is the reason why, with neural therapy, the skin is influenced in certain places.

It is impossible to explain the workings of the cabbage leaf, but we are certain of three facts:

1 It is possible to influence the affected area;
2 It produces a cleansing effect by activating the skin to eliminate poisons;
3 It creates a reflex reaction on certain reflex points on the skin.

These points however still do not satisfactorily explain the quick and effective action of the cabbage leaf.

How I hated to have to eat spinach as a child! But our ancestors knew the value of spinach and my mother made me eat it. Spinach is rich in Vitamins A, B, C, iron, calcium, phosphorous, magnesium and potassium. It stimulates the forming of red blood cells and it also cleans the bowel. Fresh spinach extract alleviates depression. It is beneficial when suffering from malfunctioning of the digestive tracts, rheumatism, arthritis, kidney stones and liver problems. It was indicated recently at a big conference in Toronto, how in natural medicine today spinach is being used for such a wide variety of health problems.

Although we regard lettuce as a common everyday vegetable, at one time it used to be difficult to obtain a lettuce, as it is a seasonal vegetable which would only grow in the hot summer months. Not only is lettuce a delicious vegetable to eat, it acts in a cooling, calming and cleansing manner. It is also rich in Vitamins A, B and C, iron, magnesium, sodium, copper and has a good blood-cleansing effect. Together with some watercress, radishes and sometimes a little celery, it makes an appetising as well as a healthy sandwich.

Since ancient times the lettuce has been known to have health properties. Earlier generations were eating it, aware of its narcotic properties, and it is also said to have been used to combat insomnia.

There are so many vegetables I could write glowing stories about, but of necessity I have to be selective. There is however one vegetable with such special properties, that I feel obliged to write in detail about it. This is the beetroot.

Oddly enough the beetroot belongs to the spinach family. It is essentially a root which is quite rich in sugar. Beetroot contains superb ingredients for the digestive system and it is of great help with constipation, bladder infections, haemorrhoids and skin diseases. But it has even more properties. This vegetable has the greatest anti-cancer organic characteristics.

I was appalled when I arrived in Scotland many years ago to see how the beetroot was being abused. Virtually the only way beetroot was eaten in this country was as pickled beetroot. Many of its health-giving properties did not survive the pickling process. Beetroot should be eaten raw or cooked in order to preserve these valuable properties. I often prescribe it as an additional product to be used by patients as a fresh beetroot drink. It is a very good medicinal remedy for the blood, as it supplies us with iron and an abundance of other minerals.

In my former residential clinic patients were served a beetroot salad every day. This contained equal amounts of raw grated beetroot and raw grated carrots, mixed with a handful of sultanas and some unsweetened apple juice. Its flavour can be enhanced by adding some Herbamare. This gives a tasty salad which is full of vitamins, minerals and trace elements to boost the immune system. It is also one of the most effective cancer preventions.

The beetroot has a very high content of potassium, copper, iron, silicone and, above all, next to the onion the beetroot has the highest silicic acid contents of Vitamin B complex. It contains betamine, a nitrogen donator/activator and stimulator of the phosphate synthesis of choline and a red fox colouring matter called cyanine. These are all very vital ingredients in the cancer therapy. Peripheral activation of cancer cells takes place when using beetroot juice combined with other activators, giving very encouraging results.

The beetroot is a natural, valuable, prophylactic and therapeutic remedy for the activation of cell respiration. The body's own defence activity centres principally around the activation of oxygen through peroxidation.

Many people do not even regard beetroot as a vegetable and I have had to instruct many patients as to its preparation. I usually give them a fairly standard recipe as it is used in The Netherlands, which is as follows:

Cook the beetroot in the skin, thus containing as many vitamins and minerals as possible. When cooked, peel off the skin, slice or grate it and mix it with some cooked and chopped onion and some dried apple. When reheating add a knob of butter and some cornflour with water to bind it. A dash of cider vinegar, a bay leaf or a pinch of ground cloves may be added.

Although the onion is not grown on a large scale in Scotland, it is generally known that it contains many health-giving ingredients. Commonly known throughout Europe, it is used as a diuretic and antiseptic and it promotes a healthy skin because it is a rich source of sulphur.

In old folklore it was often recommended to eat a raw onion because of its healthy properties and there are many varieties suitable for different purposes. Some are good for use in salads and others are better for boiling. Onion poultices on painful areas are helpful and when suffering from a cold, some onion juice mixed with honey gives great relief.

I frequently advise mothers of babies with colic and who prefer not to use any drugs to do as follows: Slice an onion, dip it into hot water and when it is lukewarm give the baby a teaspoonful of this onion water. This will relieve the colic almost at once.

If older people are bothered with digestive problems a strong onion extract in hot water can bring relief.

The onion is also rich in Vitamin C and although I am discussing the onion under the heading of vegetables, it really is as much of a seasoning as a vegetable. As it is often used in combination with other vegetables, which have been mentioned here, I decided that the onion should be included in this chapter.

In our residential clinic in The Netherlands one of our nursing sisters once had a very nasty ear infection. Her ear was swollen badly and gave her a lot of discomfort. No remedy seemed to bring relief. When one of our older colleagues visited the clinic it was discussed and he immediately made an onion poultice and placed it right on the ear and covered it with a warm, damp cloth. It seems incredible, but the abscess broke soon after and pus oozed out of it, enabling the healing process to start.

The onion is considered one of the most potent seasoning vegetables, but we should not disregard its healing potential.

Although artichokes were not often used in Britain in the olden days, they are of great value for liver and gall-bladder patients as they are rich in sulphur. In cases of liver cirrhosis due to alcohol excess we obtain excellent results by recommending the patient to eat artichokes in whatever shape or form. Dr Vogel has produced an artichoke extract called Boldocynara, which is easy to use.

In his book, *The Liver*, Dr Vogel pays a great deal of attention to the artichoke as liver patients particularly benefit from this vegetable. It promotes the production of gastric juices and liver activity. It also stimulates the flow of bile. This is one of the reasons that I sometimes recommend it for use to some people suffering migraine attacks and also to people who imbibe too much alcohol. Especially good results have been achieved with Boldocynara in the treatment of alcoholics.

Artichokes have a high inulin content, raw or cooked, and ease a craving for sweets. If one has a "sweet tooth", it will help to eat a few artichokes a week to minimise this problem.

Potatoes are not generally considered a vegetable by a Dutchman. It is of course the most used food item in The Netherlands and there is no Dutch person, man or woman, who does not sing the praises of the potato. In its role as a main course vegetable it has some wonderful properties. In Britain it has been used for centuries and especially in

Ayrshire, with its potato-growing background, the history of the potato goes back a long way.

Although a potato is easily grown, it does need some care and it is not advisable to grow potatoes in a haphazard or untidy manner. I suppose the Irish are the most famous potato growers, but I believe that the quality of the potato due to its soil dependence, is better in The Netherlands than for example in Scotland. I very often look at his face when I tell an Irishman or a Scot that a good potato grown in the clay in Zeeland is of more nutritional value than the potato here. They don't like to believe this, but I know beyond a doubt that the difference exists.

Although there are many kinds of potatoes, what is important is the category of the potato, e.g. susceptibility to drought, earliest varieties, forcing under glass, frost damage resistance, immunity to plant disease, blight resistance, common scab, highest yielders in fertile soil, etc. There are about 1600 different varieties of potato.

Very few people do not enjoy eating a potato. The potato creates a neutral reaction in the body, neither acid nor alkaline. It is also lower in protein than other vegetables. Potatoes can be eaten in many ways which makes them such a versatile ingredient in our daily diet.

Not only as a food is it a wonderful product, but I often rely on its therapeutic properties for treatment in my clinic. I advise many older arthritic patients to take the juice of one raw potato first thing in the morning, together with some mustard seeds to chew. These simple measures will improve their condition. It almost works as a filter for the acidity which is mostly present with these patients and with this inexpensive method I have seen patients almost able to get the use of their joints back again. Potato juice is most effective for uric acid and rheumatic conditions.

Not only is the juice of a potato advised for rheumatism and arthritis sufferers, it also serves as a useful remedy for stomach ulcers, eczema, chronic diarrhoea, diabetes, duodenal ulcers, psoriasis, etc. If mixed with a little milk it is ideal for swellings, bruises, inflamed muscles and inflammation of the joints. Potato poultices may also be used.

I continue to advise people to cook the potato in the skin, as we do not want to lose any of its qualities during the cooking process.

Having discussed some of the many available vegetables, we again recognise the vital force in the secrets of plant life. God has kept his promise that he would supply plenty of food for man to exist naturally. It is up to us not to spoil these gifts and to treat them with the respect they are due.

7

Fruits

WRITING ABOUT home and herbal remedies it is difficult not to mention some fruits which are widely used in this country, as fruits have also played a part in the history of natural medicine.

Let us look at the part of the apple in our daily diets because, as is often said: "An apple a day, keeps the doctor away". Apples contain more goodness than we can possibly imagine. Possibly more apples are grown in England than in Scotland and we have a choice of many varieties. An apple is regarded as a good mid-afternoon snack as it raises the blood sugar level and keeps it high. It also helps to keep hunger at bay. Nutritional researchers inform us that apples cause a slow rise in the blood sugar level, stabilising the effect of blood sugar, which together with the fibre factor helps the digestion.

Apples may be grown in a number of ways and in various places. In orchards and also on garden walls. Such are the nutritional and medicinal properties of the apple, that gardeners sometimes worked a whole day for payment of a bag of this fruit.

TRADITIONAL HOME AND HERBAL REMEDIES

A raw apple should be chewed well and eaten without removing the skin. Always wash the fruit well, because it is likely to have been sprayed with insecticides. Even if grown in our own garden, where no insecticide has been used, apples should still be properly washed as we have all heard or read of "acid rain".

The apple is very rich in vitamins, minerals and amino acids and therefore can be of such all round benefit. It is advised for constipation, intestinal infection, rheumatism, diarrhoea, hoarseness of the voice and fatigue.

I was again reminded of the value of the apple on a recent visit to Switzerland to meet my good friend Dr Vogel. After lecturing in the morning in Amsterdam, I had to continue my journey to Zurich by plane, followed by a tiring train journey. I met one of Dr Vogel's assistants and on our way to our appointment we passed one of the finest orchards in that area. As we had some time to spare, the assistant stopped and asked me to come in and look at the enormous variety of apples which were produced on this farm. I was offered one of the most delicious Cox's Pippins I have tasted and the farmer told me that I could safely eat it as he grew everything organically and would not use insecticides or pesticides.

Because of the wearying day I had behind me I had a slight headache which soon disappeared. I found this of particular interest as shortly afterwards I read that researchers had discovered that for people who suffer headaches it is of great value to regularly eat an apple. While I was eating this apple I began to feel better and the old farmer and I chatted about farming in general and fruit-farming in particular. He was a very wise and sensible person. As we all know that the origin of civilisation itself is closely linked with the decision early in mankind to settle down and work the land, we ought to be more aware of the interplay of the sun, the moon, the rain, the wind and the soil which create more or less ideal agricultural opportunities for us.

Although agriculture in the olden days may have been primitive by today's technological standards, we should never forget that fruits, and especially these fruits which should be strong and vital, deserve to be grown in a good fertile soil. Only that way will we ever be able to grow fruit which still contains its vital force. Without any question the ever-increasing world population means there is a present need for a larger food supply. If this is obtained by using chemical pesticides, fertilisers and herbicides, however, we will only receive a poorer quality food with lower nutritional value.

The mineral balance of the soil is carefully controlled by nature as to soil acidity and bacteria. We will find that the resulting fruits taste better and are of greater value. There are many ways in which the organic farmer can achieve this and good guidance should be sought. I sincerely hope that organic farming will gain in importance in the near future. With our health under constant attack from outside influences, we have to be on our guard and eat food which is grown responsibly.

Apples are such a versatile fruit and there are countless recipes in the many cookery books available on the market. We are instinctively drawn towards the apple, for it contains so much goodness.

Another fruit widely used in Britain is the pear. Pears, available in so many varieties, are rich in Vitamins A, B, C, sugar, fat, iron, calcium, phosphorous, magnesium, potassium and other minerals as well as trace elements. As the sugar of the pear is levulose, this fruit may be eaten by diabetics. A pear is not difficult to digest especially if eaten slowly. It is a laxative and is good for arthritic and high blood pressure patients.

With anaemic patients I have seen some wonderful

results when eating pears two or three times a week. Take a few dried pears which have been soaked overnight in some red wine or grapejuice. This makes a delicious dessert and enriches the blood. I advise patients who for various reasons are not in favour of blood transfusions of these simple remedies. If a patient is weak, I recommend he or she eat the above dessert daily, together with lots of fresh, green vegetables including spinach, or even a raw egg mixed with grape juice. These remedies help to keep the blood standard and if alfalfa is added we can expect good results.

If resistance to infection is poor, eat at least one pear daily, which will help to build up the natural immunity in the body. Vegetarians should also eat pears regularly. Mix pears with apples, crab-apples, lemon, grapefruit and pineapple and we have a delicious and health-giving dessert. Good fruit juices are also valuable to our health.

There are two good reasons to eat fruit regularly:
— its fibre content;
— its nutritional value.
Some fruits are more nutritious than others and a lot depends on the soil in which these fruits have been grown.

We should always remember never to eat fruit and vegetables together, as this may cause some digestive problems. This is especially true of pears. As fruit can provide a full complement of all required nutrients, we ought to get the balance right. Although it provides us with good nourishment, we have to keep the acid/alkaline balance in mind.

Plums have been grown for many years in Britain and are rich in Vitamins B and C, iron, calcium, phosphorous, magnesium and potassium. A plum is one of the finest natural laxatives and as prunes they are very often used for this purpose. Prunes are a basic ingredient in many laxatives available from the chemist.

When travelling to Lanarkshire or to the Clyde Valley it is a lovely sight to see the plum or the *Prunus Domestica* in full bloom. As it is a difficult fruit to store, we use it for jams and pies or for stewing. Prune juice is a very helpful drink for people who are allergic to milk and I have for many years taken my breakfast cereal mixed with some prune juice.

It might surprise us, but on some of the bigger estates in this country I have found figs growing on the walls of their gardens. In cases of persistent constipation a mixture of linseeds, figs and prunes has proved of great help. Figs were known in Biblical days and it is thought that Adam and Eve covered their nakedness with fig-leaves. Also in the Old Testament we read that fig-leaves were used for poultices to cure abscesses on the gums and inflammations of the mouth. King Hezekiah, the king of Judah was sick and near to death from a serious tumour. The prophet Isaiah instructed the king's attendants to make a paste of figs and spread this on the boil and the king recovered.

In the New Testament Jesus tells us the parable about the unfruitful fig tree in the book of Luke. From these stories we can deduce that the fig tree is as old as mankind and its medicinal properties known for generations.

This brings to mind an experience my mother had when she suffered a carbuncle on her neck. She had made arrangements with her doctor to have the carbuncle treated. While she was sitting in the doctor's waitingroom an old gentleman advised her to use a warm fig poultice and put it on as hot as she could possibly endure. The outcome was incredible, for shortly after my mother had put the poultice in place the carbuncle burst and a clean wound was left which soon healed. Our poor doctor was done out of a job.

Syrup of figs is of great help for chilblains, haemorrhoids, burns, abscesses and other problems.

Now we move on to a fruit which is mainly grown in greenhouses in this country — the grape. Grapes supply us with Vitamins A, B and C and also a range of proteins. They are rich in iron, phosphorous, calcium, sodium, iodine, etc. There are many cures today in which the grape features and as there are so many books available from health-food shops, dealing specifically with grape cures, I won't enlarge on them here. Grapes clear the mind, cleanse the blood and are beneficial to rheumatic, liver, gallbladder and stomach sufferers.

Although grapes are widely available in the shops today, if we intend to grow grapes in our greenhouse, good compost is a necessity. The grape is radioactive, which gives it its cleansing powers. If not home grown, it may well have been sprayed with insecticides and ought to be washed very thoroughly.

As grapes are frequently given to bedridden or hospitalised patients, most of us seem to be aware of their beneficial properties. Few people however are aware of the fact that the pips of the grape are also advantageous to our health. I frequently advise patients with arteriosclerosis or cholesterol problems to eat the pips of the grapes which should be well chewed. The pips contain ingredients which will suppress the cholesterol level. This method is particularly advisable for dysentery cases or after donating blood.

Lastly I would like to mention the tomato. Sometimes the tomato is regarded as a fruit and at other times as a vegetable. Many different opinions exist in the medical world about the tomato. Some doctors have voiced the opinion that the tomato might encourage cancer, which I think is extremely unlikely. Tomatoes have no bearing on cancer incidence. Research carried out by careful scientists has shown that cancer mortality rates are higher in those countries where the intake of protein, especially of animal protein, is excessive.

A tomato is a wonderful food, even for an arthritic patient, as long as it is a ripe tomato. The ripeness should be underlined as otherwise the tomato is too acid. To condemn the tomato is really not fair, though I am not terribly happy about the quality of tomato chutney which is used in the UK. Chutneys should be used sparingly.

Pricewise we witness locally a constant battle between the Scottish and Dutch tomatoes. Some patients ask me if the Dutch tomato is better than the Scottish one and my only answer can be that it all depends on the soil in which the tomato was grown. Today's process of growing tomatoes in water or in peat does not produce a good-quality product.

Tomatoes do not contain sodium. Among the many minerals in which they are rich is sulphur, bromine, silicone and cobalt. They also contain small amounts of Vitamin A, B and slightly more Vitamin C. Tomatoes are digested relatively quickly. They should be allowed to ripen naturally and should not be picked until they are nice and red, so that they can be eaten almost immediately.

I will repeat just once more how important a role vegetables and fruit play in our daily diet. Like each living creature, plants, foods or seeds, the human body has its own peculiar concentration of force. This force field may be compared to a natural electro-magnetic field. Any changes to this electro-magnetic field can be studied on a Kirlian photograph. This field of energy can easily be interfered with, and the balance of this energy field influenced, so we should always aim for a harmonious energy flow.

Fruit and vegetables have an invaluable energy field if grown correctly. We should not interfere with nature and we must keep these products as natural as possible.

8

Seasonings

IT IS INTERESTING to see that the Scottish Archaeological Trust has published a paper on some discoveries which were made in Perthshire. A large ditch was excavated to the east of the buildings of a Carmelite Priory, where mainly kitchen utensils were unearthed. The report shows that a soil analysis revealed the presence of medicinal herbs such as hemlock, burdock and others. It is fair to assume that these herbs were not only used, but also grown by the friars and possibly the same thing happened in other priories and abbeys. The general discussion in the booklet was about plant remains found in various parts of Perth, concluding that almost all of them had had some medicinal power attributed to them in the past. Possibly they were used for toothaches and other minor disorders.

From history we learn that the inhabitants of Perth were greatly plagued by intestinal worms and various remedies were used in order to combat this problem. I am sure that garlic — one of the finest seasonings — would have been used for this purpose. Garlic of course has a very long history, going back to the building of the great pyramids of Egypt. From old records we know that the Pharaohs were responsible for the well-being of the workforce used for the construction of these pyramids. Money was spent on garlic and other seasoning products. Where the Egyptians regarded garlic as a seasoning, the Greeks and Romans used garlic for healing purposes. In the Bible the garlic plant is mentioned as well.

Later in history we know that Napoleon provided his army with garlic to make them strong and prevent disease. Garlic, with its strong pungent flavour, however is either liked or loathed. It has a penetrating smell and produces a beautiful taste when used for culinary purposes.

Today we are eating more and more garlic and I recently read about a farm on the Isle of Wight where 120 tonnes of garlic were grown last year. Although an expensive crop to grow, increased demand today has allowed the price to come down in real terms. The medicinal use of garlic is cheap when compared to the price of drugs. As garlic has a host of medicinal qualities, not only for internal use but also for the treatment of wounds or as an antiseptic, I can well understand that in Egypt, China, Thailand and other countries, people have such a high regard for this wonderful remedy which grows freely in nature.

I have long been interested in the use of garlic because during my studies I had to help out occasionally in the pharmacy. I was always amazed to listen to the stories of our clients who purchased garlic. Customers bought garlic tablets and I was very intrigued to hear how headaches, haemorrhoids, high blood pressure, rheumatic problems and circulatory ailments were claimed to disappear. Since then I have listened with interest to the stories, mostly related by older people, about garlic's properties. When today I see garlic used medicinally in a more sophisticated form and the results obtained, I can well understand these claims.

Garlic even contains Vitamin B7, which is the anti-cancer vitamin. But it has many other properties because it activates not only the glands, but will restore the bacterial balance in the bowels and cleanse the blood. Therefore it is so useful for angina and circulatory problems. Although a lot of people do not like the smell of garlic, it does have these disinfectant powers for which it has been used over the centuries.

In present times, if garlic capsules are swallowed whole, the effects of smell and taste on the breath are minimal. It is also claimed that if a sprig of parsley is chewed raw after eating garlic, this minimises the effects on the breath. There is no doubt that although garlic originally came from Asia, it is now freely used over the whole world. It is used as a seasoning for our food and also for medicinal purposes.

Garlic milk is often taken for sciatic pain, which is very difficult to treat. Lots of people say that they have sciatica, but from experience I know that only a few people really suffer from sciatica. It reminds me of a patient who had had several acupuncture and osteopathic treatments, but still had not received any relief from the acute pain. I advised him to drink garlic milk. He did and shortly after he, at long last, was relieved from the pain.

An old lady came to see me with knee problems which, she had been told, were beyond operation. I suggested that she use garlic poultices each night, which gradually began to ease the situation.

A young girl who had been bitten by an insect also comes to mind. Unfortunately the infection would not clear up and I advised her to use garlic poultices. Luckily, this drew the poison out of the bite, proving again what a great remedy garlic is.

Garlic is rich in many minerals and particularly so in

phosphorus and bromine. A lady attended my clinic who had been suffering from sinusitus and a few minor ailments. She was delighted to tell me that she had been taking garlic, which had cleared her condition, so she too sang its praises.

When treating patients with rheumatism and arthritis, garlic destroys pathogenic and putrefactive organisms in the bowel which create toxins, causing arthritis. It also acts as a great antibiotic. This very old remedy, which is not always appreciated because of its smell, has appropriately come back into favour because of its usefulness.

Thyme is a plant which is coming more and more to the fore. It was used in the old monasteries, but perhaps more for culinary purposes than medicinally. Today it is commonly used as a seasoning. *Thymus vulgaris* is the common or garden thyme and *Thymus serpyllum* is the wild thyme or mother thyme, and there is a slight difference between the two.

In traditional history thyme has been used for many complaints. It can be used for digestive, flatulence, appetite, bronchial, insomnia and urinary problems. Whooping cough and other ailments may be treated with this herb. I have used mother thyme quite successfully for anaemia, alcoholism and even tumours. In the new cancer therapy we see that thyme is even used in injections for malignant tumours and its properties have been of tremendous help.

If we want to use this herb as a seasoning for our salad then fresh thyme should be used rather than the dried version. When used as a herb bath it is beneficial for a baby or young child who has some problems with weak lungs or is a little hoarse. Thyme is a valuable herb as its fresh extract can be used in treating facial neuralgia and even epileptic fits.

Thyme oil can be used for some skin problems. Also if

rubbed gently onto the chest it can aid attacks of bronchial asthma or emphysema.

Hyssop is a very beautiful plant and can be used not only as a seasoning, but also medicinally in various ways. It has a great disinfectant quality and sometimes it is referred to as the Biblical antibiotic. King David asked God to bathe him in hyssop so that he could come whiter than snow — in other words to cleanse him of the sins he had committed, because he was aware of the hyssop plant. God had also requested hyssop to be used in the offering of the sacrificial lamb as it was well known that this herb prevented the curdling of the blood.

Hyssop as a seasoning is very tasty. I prescribe the hyssop extract in tablet form to patients with high or low blood pressure as it is a tremendous aid to regulating this problem.

One herb which is used more in Britain than I expected it to be is parsley. It is a very old herb of medicinal value because of its contents of Vitamin C, iron and trace elements and was grown in the old monastery gardens. There are many varieties of parsley, but the most popular are green velvet and moss curl.

Because of its aroma the Greeks featured it in their banquets. The Romans also rated it highly, although in the Middle Ages it was unpopular for a while as it was thought to bring bad luck. If used in combination with some other herbs it is a very good diuretic and also a stimulant. It is good to see that it is frequently used for seasoning and the green colour makes it an attractive and decorative ingredient in our food preparation.

Although lesser known, I would like to mention the horseradish. It is such a pity that it is so often neglected because horseradish has many medicinal properties. It can aid stomach problems and it also has diuretic properties which are helpful with bladder infections. Especially the fresh horseradish can be of great value for rheumatism, gout or persistent coughing, relieving the circulation of the blood.

Slow-healing wounds may be treated with a horseradish poultice which has also relieved many a bad headache, and therefore it has many qualities similar to garlic.

As a syrup horseradish is very good to use for respiratory problems. In association with its name it has been known to be effective when administered to horses with a persistent cough.

Mint — *Mentha* is also known as wild mint, peppermint, curled mint, brandy mint, horse mint, water mint, corn mint, march mint and so on. It is good to see how frequently mint is used in the UK. According to Scottish history mint has been in use for centuries. Its virtues have influenced health for the better. Although there are many varieties of mint, they all have one thing in common and that is their flavour and aroma. If mint is cut and dried in autumn it retains its pleasant penetrating smell for many months. Mint sauce is a popular accompaniment for mutton and lamb in Britain. A few sprigs of fresh mint can be added to the water when boiling new potatoes. I would like to see mint being used more often, whether it be in its fresh form or in a medicinal mint product.

Mint in various forms may be used as an antispasmodic, carminative, stomach tonic. Peppermint tea and oil can be used for nervousness, insomnia, cramps, coughs, migraine, poor digestion, heartburn, nausea, or abdominal pains.

It is wonderful to see that mint is actually used more frequently nowadays in modern medicine. *Mentha Peperata* is used for various problems in the pharmaceutical world today. I see that even *MIMM's* advises a particular peppermint tablet for an irritated colon. This tablet contains peppermint oil, which because of its composition will effect colonic relaxation.

A Danish gentleman, Mr Obbekjaer, whose interest in herbs had been stimulated by his father, was especially intrigued by mint, a herb which was then already widely used in Denmark. He came to the conclusion after lengthy research that oil of peppermint was a most potent and beneficial preparation. He then had to find a method of administering oil of peppermint to the body. The fact that herbal preparations are frequently alcohol-based prompted him to try adding a few drops of oil of peppermint to his evening glass of wine. As mint already was popular in Denmark he had no trouble persuading his neighbours and friends to assist him in his experiments. A general improvement of health was reported. Some had experienced improved digestion and others reported improvement in their circulation, eyesight, rheumatic or arthritic pains and even migraines diminished.

However, Mr Obbekjaer became concerned that too much wine as a carrier for the oil of peppermint might have obvious side-effects. He was aware that when athletes want to increase their energy output quickly, they use glucose, dextrose or honey and so he began compounding a mixture of powdered dextrose and oil of peppermint into a tablet. The beneficial effects remained unchanged so he began to distribute this product. Due to the improvement noticed by those using Mr Obbekjaer's tablets, his fame spread from village to village. Soon he was unable to cope with the production. He arranged for his tablets to be produced on a large scale and to be marketed all over Denmark. The fame of his product has now spread to many countries, largely due to personal recommendation.

The 84-year-old Mr Obbekjaer attributes his health and longevity to the continued use of oil of peppermint. Letters arrive at Mr Obbekjaer's and his world-wide agents, testifying to the beneficial results experienced by many on taking Obbekjaer's oil of peppermint, which is now obtainable in powdered and tablet form from most health-food shops.

I have used this peppermint product in my practice for a number of years and was delighted when a doctor of medicine recently referred with great respect to this peppermint cure. He regards the treatment with peppermint oil to be absolutely free of side-effects and considers it beneficial for the various diseases and ailments listed.

As stated before, I am delighted to see some of the old and tried herbal remedies coming back into fashion. These herbs should not be restricted to use in the kitchen. Used medicinally some of them are now available in tablet form.

I now turn to a preparation which is as much a seasoning for salads as it is a herbal remedy. In Britain in the seventeenth and eighteenth century it was known as milk whey or the whey of the milk. On 30 May 1768 William Cullen wrote in the *History of Scottish Medicine* about the great value of the then known whey cure for the digestion. Today there is a product called Molkosan, produced by Dr Vogel, which is both useful as a salad dressing and as a medicine. It is known as The Swiss Whey-Cure and is beneficial when dealing with obesity, circulation, congestion, metabolism, intestinal ailments, gastric acid secretion and diabetes.

Writing about Molkosan reminds me of the time I approached my bank manager for an overdraft to expand my clinic in The Netherlands. Unfortunately the bank manager had a mild form of diabetes and was advised to take tablets, but would have to resort to insulin injections if his condition deteriorated. He then asked me if I could advise him on his health problems. I used some herbal remedies, a tincture of the extract of walnut tree leaves, and I suggested that he daily drink the whey of the milk, which is available in Molkosan. Within six weeks his blood sugar level was back to normal. His doctor advised him that there was no further need of medication as he was completely clear of diabetes. Luckily I received the overdraft I so very much needed and we still remain very good friends. This episode stimulated his interest in natural medicine so that on retiral he became chairman of a naturopathic group in The Netherlands.

Molkosan can also be used as a gargle and is excellent for clearing mouth ulcers, especially in youngsters who are taking too much sugar or sweets. If dabbed on, it will greatly assist the clearing of athlete's foot and slow-healing wounds. It can also be used to clear skin disorders. The concentrated milk whey, with its natural lactic acid and disinfectant properties, has been of great help for all these ailments.

Last but not least there is Herbamare — a herbal seasoning — produced by Dr Vogel. Herbamare is made from fresh — not dried — herbs. It contains chives, basil, marjoram, watercress and other kinds of cress, rosemary, thyme, parsley and kelp. These herbs are cultivated in the clean, fresh mountain air of Switzerland, far from industry and large population centres. The herbs are grown organically without the use of chemical pesticides and fertilisers.

The fresh herbs are combined with real, wet sea salt and allowed to steep. This permits the salt to extract the flavour from the herbs and at the same time to preserve the natural antibiotic qualities of the parsley and cress. Herbamare can be used in the kitchen in the preparation of raw or cooked vegetables, stews, gravies, soups, rice and all forms of salads. It is available from most health-food shops.

9

Cereals

WHEN LECTURING I always stress the value of cereals, so I am pleased to have this opportunity to write about them. Cereals are of great nutritional value if used correctly. Unfortunately the traditional breakfast porridge has largely disappeared from our tables. If we think that Scottish oats are considered to be the best in the world, I can only be grateful that there are still some wise people who give their families porridge oats for breakfast.

Not only are the oats — *Avena sativa* — a wonderful food, they are of tremendous nutritional value to the nerves. With great pleasure I have witnessed in Switzerland that when the harvest is ready, the Swiss farmer cuts the tops off the oats and soaks these in some alcohol, usually some brandy. Thus he obtains the finest tranquiliser we can find, and one which can be used safely by all members of the family.

Oats, or *Avena savita* have over the years been of great value. It is such a pity that the use of oats as a natural remedy was lost on recent generations. *Avena sativa* as a homoeopathic remedy is recommended for hyper-active and highly strung children. Oatmeal gruel or porridge can help a nervous stomach.

During its growth when it is tall, it has some remarkable healing powers. When the stalks of the oats are green the Avenen content is at its highest level. Avenen is a marvellous nutrient for the cells of the nervous system. It is no wonder that horses who receive their strength and their health from eating oats, thrive on it. It is just as important for horses as it is for human beings to have a well-balanced diet.

This reminds me of a very difficult horse I once treated. The horse had a nervous disposition and was extremely difficult to handle. His owner approached a good friend of mine who put her in touch with me. She told me that when entering the horse's loose box in the morning he would be standing there covered in a white lather of sweat as if he had been galloping for hours. The vet was unable to improve the situation with any of his medicines and wondered if there was a future for the poor animal. I recommended some homoeopathic remedies without any result. We discussed the feeding or the diet of the horse and I was told that it was eating a large quantity of barley. I suggested feeding the horse increased quantities of oats. In a few weeks' time the horse's temperament changed and he became more manageable.

Eventually the owner was able to report to me that the excessive sweatings of the horse had stopped. A few months later she phoned me to report the progress of the horse. She was delighted to tell me that all was well and she was able to ride him every week in her new role as joint master of the local hunt. This goes to show how fantastic oats are, even for horses.

One day the headmaster of one of the local schools approached me about one of his pupils. This poor girl was under a lot of strain and she had always been a hyper-active child. Luckily, *Avena sativa* helped to sort out her difficulties and she was able to continue with her usual studies. No further behavioural problems were apparent.

Scottish porridge oats are a good start to the day for their digestive and structural muscle building properties. Oats contain iron, copper trace elements and even more calcium than is found in wheat or rice. Oats may certainly be used in many forms and should not be absent from our breakfast table. In olden days it was said that when the shepherds cooked their porridge, they made a quantity sufficient to last them for a few days. After they had had their breakfast, the remainder of the porridge would be poured into a drawer. When cold and set, it was easily cut into squares and these portions could be taken into the hills to sustain them on their long vigils looking after their sheep.

In bygone days most of the hay-making work was done in dusty and hot conditions. Water was brought to the men in the fields and to this was added some oatmeal. The drink was very thirst-quenching and gave them the additional energy required to enable them to work from dawn till dusk. Oats were bruised before being fed to cattle and sheep. Farmers were not wasteful and the straw which was left, was used for other purposes.

We now arrive at another cereal — wheat. Wheat and rice are the most widely grown foods in the world though wheat is the more popular in the West. What has happened to our wheat during the years of agricultural development? If it were once again grown organically, we would have a good strong wheat which would be more beneficial to us all and there would be less risk of allergic reactions.

I often state in lectures that our energy has never been attacked as much as it is in this day and age, for food is our source of energy. Wheat in its original form was the finest food available as promised by God in the Bible, and was one of the most valuable food products in our daily diet. Unfortunately in our efforts to increase food production the original properties of wheat have been changed drastically. This has interfered with our immune system and the result is an increasing number of people who suffer from allergies.

Often patients come to me with skin problems which are simply the result of a wheat allergy. Over the years the need for increased food production has resulted in the agricultural scientists working towards an increased crop. Due to this, the wheat grain has a vastly increased number of chromosomes which results in allergic reactions in some people. If organically grown grains were used for our bread and cakes, they would contain more nutritional value and there would be fewer allergies.

It would be much better if in the milling process grinding stones of different composition were used. These would add many minerals to the flour. The Mexican Indians use soft limestone for grinding the corn for their tortillas, which add calcium to their diets.

To summarise:

— Wheat is acid forming;

— Barley is high in calcium, which is easy on the digestive system;

— Oats are rich in silicone, necessary for the brain;

— Rye produces muscle and is rich in Vitamin E, phosphorous, magnesium, silicone and the EFA's (Essential Fatty Acids);

— Rice builds the body, bones, teeth and contains ten times more minerals than any other organic cereal;

— Millet is alkaline-forming and rich in BS lecithine and several amino acids.

So we arrive at millet, which was already in use in Biblical days and is an acid/alkaline balancer for other cereals. It is richer in Vitamins B15 and B17 than other cereals and millet does not ferment in the stomach as rapidly as wheat does. In northern China, unexpectedly, millet is used more than rice. It was also a staple food in the American diet during the last century. The Hunzas, with their reputation for good health and longevity, use millet and so do the Russians.

Recently I attended a lecture where it was stated that millet contains mineral matter which enables alkalines to neutralise acid forming constituents. A doctor from Yale University claims millet to be a complete food substance containing vitamins, minerals, protein and lecithine. Therefore it helps prevent the accumulation of cholesterol on the inner lining of the arteries.

Bread baked with millet is not considered to produce a very tasty loaf. However, once, when I was lecturing in Canada at a big health conference, a lady was kind enough to send to my room some loaves which were known in Canada as millet bread and they did taste extremely good. On checking with her, I discovered that the bread did not contain any wheat, but that some rye had been added. This combination of cereals makes a delicious bread which produces large amounts of energy to fuel the body.

Dr Moerman from The Netherlands developed a new cancer therapy, which largely featured millet. For his research he studied pigeons because of the similarity between their metabolism and the human metabolic system. Pigeons exist mainly on millet and when their diet was altered their health deteriorated. This factor he took into account when developing his therapy which has been of such tremendous help to so many people.

Rye is often condemned because of its acid-forming qualities. Arthritic people should not eat too much of it. Foods with alkaline-forming properties, especially those rich in sodium, potassium, calcium, magnesium and iron, should be taken in combination with other foods to find the correct acid/alkaline balance. Many people who are allergic to wheat are able to eat rye, although some of them have to learn to eat it — it is an acquired taste.

My health deteriorated badly as a result of severe food shortages during the Second World War. One of the first foods which became available after the war was rye bread, which had a slightly sour taste. This put me back on the road to good health. However, dark rye bread should be well chewed and not eaten in excess.

Barley, although a great source of nutrition, should also be taken in moderate amounts. Barley water mixed with milk will ease throat, stomach and intestinal problems as it has a soothing effect. Fevers can be reduced by the administration of barley water. Traditionally, barley is a main ingredient in scotch broth which is a nutritional food in itself.

In the United States I discovered a bread which is called the Ezekiel bread. This is the bread which is mentioned in the Bible in Ezekiel 4: verse 9, which consisted of six ingredients: wheat, barley, beans, lentils, millet and spelt. To make this bread the ingredients should be boiled quickly, after which the slow cooking should continue in a hay box, thus preserving the nutrients. If these ingredients were pre-soaked the goodness would be lost in the water.

The next cereal on my list is buckwheat, which is widely used in some countries. The Greeks use it as an ingredient in one of their national dishes. Whole buckwheat may be cooked in a similar way to rice. Some nutritionists recommend buckwheat for the relief of high blood pressure. It has been advised that the older generation particularly use brown rice or buckwheat as both cereals are low in protein and salt.

My good friend Dr Ann Wigmore, the founder and

director of the Research Institute for Useful Living recently said: "It is not the food in your life which brings health, it is the life in your food that really counts." She is an authority on the sprouting of grains and seeds and has published many papers on the subject. She is an excellent example of her own teaching. In her book *Be your own doctor* she describes different methods of food preparation to retain its energy-giving substances and this has proved of benefit to many people.

Rice is the last cereal I will write about in detail. As I mentioned in my book on nervous disorders, rice is of tremendous value and it saddens me that it is not eaten more frequently in this country. The Chinese are well aware of the beneficial properties of wholegrain brown rice as they know the importance of the yin and yang balance in their diet.

Dr Anthony Sattilaro, although over 50, looks a picture of health. It is hard to believe that two years ago he was dying of cancer. A medical doctor himself, his cancer was diagnosed as stage 4 prostatic carcinoma, which had metastasized (spread of cancer cells to other parts of the body) from the prostate to the bones. Tests showed the cancer to be pervasive throughout the body, in the skull, the right shoulder, probably the sternum, the left sixth rib and the genital region. Surgeons had removed some cancerous tumours but all to no avail. While travelling one day he picked up a couple of hitch-hikers who tried to convince him that the macrobiotic diet would cure cancer. Dr Satillaro was sceptical, but as he had nothing to lose, he gave it a try. After two weeks his pain had diminished to such an extent that he could reduce his drug intake. After thirteen months on the diet the cancer specialists found no trace of cancer in his body.

As the macrobiotic diet centres around wholegrain brown rice, my recommendations that rice should be used more often should not come as a surprise. Rice has numerous qualities, especially if we use the wholegrain brown rice. Unfortunately the bleached white rice is of little nutritious value. As mentioned earlier, when as a child I had a stomach disorder, my mother would give me some rice with blackcurrant juice or jelly and the problem would soon be resolved.

If we look at the rice grain we see that the inner kernel consists of starch. This starch or carbohydrate is a high calorific or heat-producing food. It would be unwise to dispose of that starch because it contains the elements we need. Other vital constituents of the rice grain are fats, proteins, phosphates and vitamins. If we cook wholegrain brown rice properly, it is absolutely untrue that it is difficult to digest.

The Dutch doctor Eykman discovered that the rice bran alone had the properties to cure beri-beri. Fortunately it is helpful for a number of other conditions. Natural brown rice contains nine and a half times more minerals than polished, refined rice when cooked properly. A wholegrain brown rice diet can minimise the effects of high blood pressure. In China where I studied acupuncture and where rice is used as a daily food, I did not see the high blood pressure problems we have in our western world today. Rice contains all the vitamins, minerals and trace elements we need. It is a delicious food and extremely versatile, if only we remember to cook it properly. In this respect I will repeat the rice recipe which I so often advise.

Put the desired quantity of rice into a casserole or oven-proof dish. Pour over boiling milk or, preferably, water. Have the oven pre-heated at the highest temperature, and place the dish of rice in the oven for 10 or 15 minutes. Switch the oven off and leave the rice inside for five to six hours. Cut up some vegetables — parsley, chicory, celery and cress, for example — and mix through the rice with a little garlic salt. When required heat through.

With all cereals it is of major importance that we know how to use and respect them.

10

Home Remedies

AS I REACH the closing stages of this book on herbal and plant remedies, I most definitely must include a section on home remedies used over many generations. Although these home remedies may be of little scientific use, they have most certainly proven their worth. We may shrug our shoulders and consider such remedies useless, yet at one time or another they were invaluable.

Distance was once a major problem for people living in remote areas. They would sometimes be totally isolated due to heavy snowfalls or flooding of the roads. Without modern communications it was impossible to contact a doctor in times of illness. Natural healing methods, passed on from generation to generation, would then be used by parents and grandparents alike. Their instinct for self-preservation would be so great that fevers, influenza and even broken bones were treated successfully, using methods which were passed down by word of mouth.

There was undoubtedly a very effective range of home treatments and because these were based on a sound principle of healing, looking at illness as a whole, remarkable recoveries took place. The drug-less programme of natural healing flourished until industrialisation caused many natural skills to be lost. Attitudes changed and the desire for speedier results gained momentum. However, the wheel is turning again — back to natural treatment.

Medical practitioners are in such demand that people again try to help themselves with minor problems. Home treatments were once often used to overcome aches and pains, colds and influenza. Inflammatory conditions could be reduced and exercising mental control over pain was practised more in those days than at present.

An estimated thirteen million prescriptions for strong painkillers are written out each year in Britain and one-quarter of all the money spent on over-the-counter remedies goes to pain-relieving drugs. These are undoubtedly effective for many people, for others however they are only marginally effective or completely ineffective and may result in vomiting, diarrhoea or internal bleeding. We should always be aware of the risk of possible side-effects. Herbal remedies and home treatments may very occasionally produce some adverse reactions and it must be stressed that common sense should always prevail, but the risk with these remedies is infinitely smaller than with drug treatments. Our stomachs are designed to receive food and drink; oral medicines are not always the logical solution when suffering from localised problems.

Medical research involves astronomical amounts of money and once more I state that it would be to our advantage if only a fraction of this were spent on researching some of these old forms of natural treatment.

Dr John Hughes Bennett, who lived from 1812-1875, realised the therapeutic value of cod liver oil. In 1845 he published papers on a case of leucocythaemia which was treated successfully with cod liver oil. Widely used by the population of fishing villages, cod liver oil became established as one of the finest remedies. Today in the development of evening-primrose oil, cod liver oil is used as a neuro-transmitter with excellent results. The value of these natural home treatments depends largely on the understanding of what is happening in our body. Each individual practitioner must decide on a specific course of action when the cause of the problem is discovered.

Again, every time I travel through the beautiful little country village of Eaglesham in Scotland, I am reminded of the fact that in the history of this little village during an epidemic of smallpox, many home remedies were used successfully.

We are privileged that such remedies have been preserved and handed down to us to work with and to experience their beneficial value. A positive approach is essential and first of all we should be aware of the nourishment our bodies require. A well-balanced diet of fruits, vegetables, nuts and grains is necessary, as are exercise, rest and oxygen. We need to respect Nature's laws, which are the laws of God. Sometimes on my travels I look at the environment, the junk foods, the poisoned soil, the abuse of alcohol and tobacco and the excessive use of drugs. We urgently need to change and ask ourselves whether or not we have reached the point of no return.

In the book *Nature Hits Back*, written in 1936 by Dr MacPherson Lawrie, I read the following quotation: "Those whom the Gods wish to destroy, they first make mad." He comments: "Today man makes his brain his God and this God begins to undermine his sanity." Even in those days it was already realised that we are part of nature and that by attacking instead of supporting our health in various ways, we destroy those properties which could be of such value. I am grateful when I meet people who are prepared to listen and learn. Even those people with severe health problems, who realise the benefits of a well-balanced diet and the use of those things God had entrusted us with.

Back in the fourteenth century the famous Dr Paracelsus said that our fields and mountains function according to the process of chemistry. So much is created in nature for us to take advantage of.

The question whether home remedies work remains. They work very well when used properly. Many remedies which have been used consistently across cultures and centuries surprise modern pharmacists with their efficacy. While modern drugs will remove symptoms, they often do not cure the cause. Herbal or home remedies usually act in a more gentle manner, but are of more value in the long run.

Home remedies tickle our curiosity and are sometimes referred to as old wives' superstitions. We tend to believe that they are all right for uncivilised peoples, but they have been a blessed aid in many illnesses and diseases. I hope that many readers will be inspired to use some of these traditional herbal and home remedies in the future. At the many lectures I have attended throughout the world, I have benefited greatly from the questions asked by people in the audience or from their answers where my knowledge fell short.

What is the point of goat's milk? There is little point trying to explain this scientifically. An old lady of nearly ninety told me that if goats eat certain herbs and weeds, they are able to produce milk of a quality which may be used in the treatment of otherwise incurable eczema.

Sheep eat cotton grass (*Euriophorum augustifolium*) because they instinctively realise the benefits this contains for them. At one time it was thought that the long and healthy lives of the Balkan shepherds could be attributed to their regular use of yoghurt. Now, however, it appears that it is not so much the yoghurt, but the milk of which it is made.

Often in our ignorance we dismiss these old remedies out of hand. Recently during a lecture to a group of medical doctors and students I noticed that their questions implied ignorance and incredulity. With our modern science and technology we tend to overlook the simple and proven methods. In this lecture I quoted the words which Robert Burns, the world-renowned Scottish poet, wrote to his contemporary, Dr Moore: "It ever was my opinion that the mistakes and blunders both in a rational and religious point of view, of which we see thousands daily guilty are owing to their ignorance of themselves. To know myself has been all along my constant study. I weighed myself alone; I balanced myself with others; I watched every means of information, to see how much ground I occupied as a man and as a poet; I studied assiduously NATURE's design in my formation — where the lights and shades in my character were intended."

From numerous sources over the years I have collected many genuine home remedies. On the following pages you might find some remedies you will use yourself and others which you will read and wonder about. I promise you, though, that these are all genuine, however unusual or unappealing they might seem. The reader may find some of these remedies hard to understand and appreciate in modern times. It should however be noted that many of the remedies have been passed down from generation to generation by word of mouth. Others have been written down and where appropriate the original text has been used.

Abscesses

— Abscesses may be successfully treated with Tincture of Ivy.

— Abcesses on fingers, i.e. whitlows, are simple to cure by using the following method: Soak finger or toe in warm water — 100°F or 38°C. Continue to do this three times daily for one hour at a time. Alternatively, soak finger in hot water to which some bicarbonate of soda has been added.

Aches and Pains

— An ointment for all kinds of aches: Take gander's fat, the fat of a male cat and red boar's fat and three drams of blue wax, watercress, wormwood, the red strawberry plant and primrose. When boiled in pure spring water, stuff the gander with this and roast it at a distance from the fire. The grease issuing from the gander should be kept carefully in a pot, which is a valuable ointment for all kinds of aches in man's body. It is like a salve which was formerly made by Hippocrates.

— Steep marigolds in good cider vinegar and frequently wash the affected parts with this liquid. This will afford speedy relief.

— Take half a pound of tar and half a pound of tobacco and boil these down separately till a thick substance has been obtained. Then simmer them together. Spread this substance onto a plaster and apply this to the affected parts and it will bring immediate relief.

— Roast some salt in the oven until it is the colour of roasted coffee. Dissolve a soupspoonful in a glass of water and swallow.

— For neuralgia pains use field thistles to make a tea and also a poultice. The leaves are macerated and used as a poultice on the affected parts, while a small quantity of the same is boiled and reduced by half. A small wineglass of this decoction should be drunk before each meal.

— An old French peasant remedy against rheumatic pains:

Marinate four large heads of garlic in four-fifths of a pint of brandy for 10 days. Take half a teaspoon in half a glass of water first thing every morning.

— Bathing in bay leaves:
Eight tablespoons of crushed bay leaves
1 pint of boiling water
1 pint of cider vinegar
Place the bay leaves in a heat-resistant container and pour over the boiling water. Cover and infuse for 30 minutes. Add vinegar and leave for one hour. Strain and bottle. Pour a pint of this infusion into the bathwater and relax for 15 to 20 minutes in the bath. It will ease the aches and pains of a hectic and tiring day.

— For a sore lip chew tormentil.

— Slippery Elm poultice: Combine charcoal and slippery elm in equal quantities. Both should be in a dry powder form so they can be mixed with warm water into a paste. Use this poultice for gangerous sores or inflamed areas of the body, especially glands. It is also effective if used internally.

Acne

— One litre of stinging nettle tea should be taken during the day. Treatment to be continued till complaint clears.

— Two tablespoons of blackstrap molasses daily.

— A grape diet for the duration of ten days. Three times daily at mealtimes eat only grapes. Drink plenty of water. Have an enema twice daily made up of two pints of warm water. Every second day stand in the bath and wet the body and rub salt over the wet skin as vigorously as possible. Afterwards wash the body down with cold water.

Anaemia

— Take large quantities of green salad, stinging nettle

juice, spinach, vegetable juice (especially beetroot and carrot juice) daily.

— Eat pears which are dried without sulphur or other chemicals and soak these overnight in a sweet red wine. Take this three times per week.

— Three times a week take a raw egg beaten in some fresh grape juice. Eat lots of raw beetroot and carrots daily.

— Eat germinated wheat daily.

Appetite

To create an appetite:

— Chew a piece of rhubarb an hour before dinner.

— Drink a small glass of bitters one hour before dinner.

— One hour before dinner suck two or three ginger lozenges.

— Drink half a pint of nettle tea mixed with some Centaurium one hour before dinner daily.

Arthritis

— Drink cabbage juice daily.

— Daily drink raw potato juice with three to four mustard seeds.

— Use blackstrap molasses daily.

— Press the juice of three grapefruits , three oranges and three lemons. Take two ounces of cream of tartar and two ounces of epsom salts and dissolve in one pint of boiling water. Grind the fruit pulp, seeds and skin in a container and scald with one quart of boiling water. Mix fruit juice with the pulp and let it stand overnight. Extract juice from pulp and add tartar and salts combination. Mix and then bottle. Take three ounces every morning before breakfast.

After this course a total acid-free diet is recommended.

— The cod liver oil cure by Dale Alexander:

1 To achieve the best results, take your cod liver oil mini milkshake one hour before breakfast. If more convenient, you may drink the mixture just before bedtime — at least four hours after your evening meal (or last food).

2 It is important to use a four or five ounce screwtop jar. If you use a larger jar, more of the oil will be left clinging to the inside surface of the jar and your body will receive a lesser amount.

3 To mix and emulsify the cod liver oil with whole milk is a simple procedure. Pour two ounces of whole milk into a screwtop jar. The jar should be large enough to hold four to five ounces of liquid.

4 Add one tablespoon of cod liver oil. Shake vigorously for about fifteen seconds. The cod liver oil mini milkshake will then become foamy. Drink the mixture immediately.

5 Do not take any food after this oil mixture for at least an hour.

6 If you are allergic to milk, or do not prefer it, you may use two ounces of fresh strained orange juice to prepare the mixture. However, cod liver oil is more effective and works faster when it's mixed with milk.

7 Cod liver oil capsules should not be used as substitution for the oil. The contents of the capsules is quickly captured by the liver, since gelatin promotes digestion, and the skin linings are denied proper lubrication.

8 After a while you can start to cut down on the use of the mixture. When it is noticed that dryness of hair or scalp has been corrected, or when a normal supply of wax returns to the ears, cut down on the cod liver oil intake.

9 Do not stop taking cod liver oil suddenly. At first, consume the mixture every other morning, instead of daily. Continue to follow this plan for approximately six months. Then it can be cut down to once a week.

If your gallbladder has been removed or if experiencing gallbladder trouble, only use one teaspoon of cod liver oil and take it on alternate days.

Other people who should deviate from the above rules are those suffering from ailments like high blood pressure, heart disease and diabetes. They may not assimilate oils very quickly and should take cod liver oil every other night or twice a week.

Those with eczema, psoriasis, dermatitis, any kind of ulcer or skin irritation due to nervous conditions should use only whole milk in their mixture as anyone with the ailments mentioned above is often allergic to the citric acid and fruit sugar of the orange.

Asthma

— Wash the head in cold water every morning and take a cold bath every two weeks.

— Use a decoction of liquorice, which will relieve the symptoms.

— Take half a pint of tar water twice a day.

— For two weeks live mainly on boiled carrots.

— Steep cabbage in a good quantity of water and when totally sodden wring the juice out. Drink this juice first thing in the morning and last thing at night.

— Mix two ounces of honey with one ounce of castor oil. Take a teaspoon of this mixture every morning and evening.

— Take a daily dose of equal quantities of castor oil and vinegar.

Athlete's Foot

— Dab daily with milk whey or Molkosan. Afterwards rub with St John's wort oil.

TRADITIONAL HOME AND HERBAL REMEDIES

Bad Breath

— Use oil of peppermint.
— Drink daily sage and wormwood tea.
— Drink half a teaspoon of kaolin in warm water.
— Drink nettle beer.
— Drink the water in which a mixture of barley, figs, raisins and liquorice has been soaked.

Bed Sores

— Rub the affected areas with Sunlight soap and dry off with a hairdryer or in front of the fire. Afterwards use St John's wort oil or powder.

Bedwetting

— Rub bladder area with comfrey extract with a circular movement while bending the right groin.
— Daily drink lady's-mantle tea.
— Bedwetting in children is often the result of a nervous or highly strung disposition. It can also be caused by the irritation of high acidity of a body in a fairly toxic state. Epsom salts will take care of both problems. Bathe the child each night in a bath with some Epsom salts added to the bath-water and this will relax and settle the nerves and draw off the acidity. This will ensure a dry bed unless there is another cause for the problem. Do not however expect immediate results.

Boils

— Take one tablespoonful of equal amounts of sulphur and treacle each night and each morning, which will cleanse the blood.
— The skin of a boiled egg is the best remedy for a boil.

Carefully remove the shell from the egg, wet the skin and apply to the boil. It draws out matter and relieves the soreness.
— Use warm bread poultices for the draining of boils.
— Spread honey on boils to ease the pain.
— Clean boils with marigold extract.
— Place a cabbage-leaf poultice on the boil and bandage this in place.
— Spread warm boiled linseeds onto the boil.

Bronchitis

— User Masterwort tea daily.
— Apply a hot mustard poultice to the chest at bed-time.
— Use a hot kaolin poultice on the chest and leave on all night.

Bruises

— Use arnica internally and externally.
— Drink Hamamelis tea daily.
— Boil hard groundsel of elderflower and wormwood together and then apply to the bruise.
— Dissolve a teaspoon of camphor in half a pint of olive oil to make a liniment. Rub this well into the affected parts twice daily.
— Use cabbage-leaf poultices.
— Beat three or four eggwhites and mix with thirty grams of pulverised Eucalyptus leaves or pine needles. Spread this paste on the affected areas and bandage with cotton strips and an elasticated bandage. If necessary this may be repeated two days later. Results will show surprisingly soon.

Burns

— Take a quarter pound each of beeswax, burgundy pitch, white pitch and rosin; half a pound of mutton tallow; a quarter pint of goose oil and one-eighth of a pint of tar. Mix and melt these ingredients together and use this mixture as a salve for burns.

— Apply the smooth side of the peach-tree leaves to the skin and bind them on.

— Carefully peel and core an apple and beat it with salad oil until it is a soft mixture. Spread this paste on to the burn and when it has dried apply a fresh poultice. If the skin of the burn, however, is broken there is nothing in nature to take out the fire.

— An old Irish recipe: To heal a burn without leaving a scar, take sheep's suet and the bark of the elder-tree. Boil both together and the ointment will cure a burn without leaving a mark.

— Take the root of the docken plant and boil it together with a little fresh butter. Apply this mixture as a dressing on a bandage.

— Spread fish oil on a burn.

— Slice some mushrooms and spread the slices over the affected area.

— Immediately apply peat soot from the chimney to a burn. Although this is a very sore remedy, it is most effective.

— To spread eel fat onto a burn is very good.

— Spread some honey over burns.

— Immediately immerse the affected part in cold water and then cover with a poultice of slippery elm. Apply St John's wort oil afterwards.

Chilblains

— Take footbaths in a hot potato concoction or in an oak bark concoction.

— Roast onions and turnips, mix with some turpentine and spread this paste on the affected areas.

— Take pretty thick, fresh cut parings from turnips and hold them to the fire till crisp. Then apply these strips to unbroken blisters, as hot as can be endured and keep them on for a competent time. Repeat if required. They will relieve the discomfort without breaking the blisters.

— Wear flannel sock or socks of chamois leather to prevent chilblains.

— Take the itch out of chilblains by rubbing them frequently with a raw onion.

— For the soothing of painful and unbroken chilblains: Make a concoction of celery stalks by boiling nine ounces of stalks in one-and-three-quarter pints of water for fifteen minutes. Allow it to cool and dip the affected parts in it for five minutes. Or bathe the affected parts with a concoction of walnut leaves.

— When going to bed at night, put hands and feet in very hot water and then dry them thoroughly with an old linen cloth, patting them so that the linen removes all the moisture from the pores. Put your hands and feet right up to the fire for a while. Then make an oatmeal poultice, just like porridge without salt. Spread this on the areas and leave till morning. Then make another oatmeal poultice and put this on without washing the feet and hands. In the evening again wash hands and feet in hot water and repeat the process. Continue with this method for a week and it will cure chilblains.

Circulation

— Cold Dip: This exercise has to be done each morning on

rising and each night on retiring. Place a basin of cold water and a towel at the side of the bed. When getting up in the morning place both feet into the water. Count till ten and remove both feet onto the towel to dry. Exercise the toes as if trying to pick up a marble. Do this 10-30 times. Carry out the same procedure when retiring at night. You will find that your feet will be as warm as toast when you go to bed. The importance of this exercise is that it should be done for a minimum of sixty days if you want to feel the benefit.

— Drink daily a mixture of St John's wort and arnica.

— On seeing the first St John's wort flower of the season a Gaelic verse should be recited to the effect of:

> A flower of St John
> without wanting or longing
> won't you grant me my first wish.

— To stimulate the body's defence system a hot and cold foot-bath is quite effective. Use a hot only footbath in treating colds, but sometimes a warming and stimulating process gives better results. This is especially true when the body has succumbed to a cold as a result of being very exhausted.

— Circulation increased — swelling relieved — cleans out clogged veins and arteries! When cold water strikes the foot, the blood in that extremity tends to be hurried up the leg by the contraction of the small blood vessels stimulated by the cold. Immediately, a fresh supply of blood pours in to take the place of the blood which had been flowing sluggishly. The tissues are revitalised by the life giving oxygen and cell food supplied by the fresh blood.

Try applying cold water to the ankles which are swollen by the end of the day.

What applies to the foot is equally true of other parts of

the body. We all know that a quick dash of cold water to the face brings a healthy glow to the skin. The same goes for the legs, chest, back or arms — wherever cold water is used, it brings a new rush of fresh blood.

Colds and coughs

— Balm for a sore throat: Mix one ounce of marsh-mallow root and one ounce of honey in four-fifths of a pint of water. Gargle well with the liquid several times a day.

— Gargle with salt and water — half a teaspoon to a glass of warm water.

— Gargle with the juice of a lemon in a glass of warm water.

— Eat dry sugar.

— Drink a cup of hot water with a spoonful of treacle before going to bed.

— Sip onion water throughout the day.

— Take one teaspoonful of sugar with three drops of eucalyptus oil to stop coughing at night.

— For a sore throat place a sweaty sock round the throat at night.

— Take a dessertspoonful of blackcurrant jam in a cup of hot water at night.

— A very old colds remedy: Use black sheep's wool and butter. Or use black sheep's wool, olive oil and eggs.

— Take sage leaves, rub them and apply them to the nostrils in the morning.

— Boil holly bark in goat's milk and drink this while still warm.

— Take a quarter of a pint of horehound water, a quarter of a pint of coltsfoot water, a pound of stoned raisins, which should be pounded well. Mix these ingredients together and then set them on the fire. Boil them like marmalade. Add two ounces of honey and one spoonful of mustard and let it simmer a while. Pot this mixture and take as much as the quantity of a walnut first thing in the morning and last thing at night.

— For catarrh, drink Epsom salts dissolved in warm water.

— Take one cup of honey, half a cup of vinegar and some cayenne pepper.

— Infuse three drachms of garlic and half an ounce of mustard seed into two pints of white wine. Let this stand covered for a week and then drink a glass of this as often as you please.

— If suffering from a cold blister, rub a slug on it.

— Take some buttonwood, white oak and white ash barks in equal quantities, boil in water and sweeten with honey. Take one tablespoon three times a day.

— Use warm compresses on the chest.

— To stop a consumptive cough keep a little stick of liquorice shaved like horseradish between the cheek and gums when lying down.

— Eat preserved walnuts.

— Drink water whitened with oatmeals four times a day.

— For a tickling cough: keep a piece of barley sugar or sugar candy constantly in the mouth.

Colic

— For babies: Slice an onion and dip it in hot water. Give the baby half a teaspoonful of this onion water a few times a day.

— Take the husks of green beans and distill them. Take the water thereof, add a little stale ale and sip until the colic pains have eased.

— Eat a gallon or more of chicken broth.

— Take one eighth of a pint of good rye whiskey and a pipe full of tobacco. Put the whiskey into a bottle and smoke the tobacco. Blow the smoke into the bottle, shake it and drink it.

— Take a white clay pipe which has turned blackish from smoking, pound it into a fine powder and chew this powder.

Constipation

— Half a pound of raisins, half a pound of dates, half a pound of figs, two ounces of powdered senna, one ounce of powdered sulphur and half an ounce of powdered ginger. Mix powdered ingredients together, put all the fruit through the mincer twice or through a liquidiser, then blend it well with the powdered ingredients. If too dry, add a teaspoon of glycerine. Take a small portion at bedtime.

— One tablespoon of cornmeal stirred up in sufficient cold water to drink easily. This should be drunk in the morning immediately on rising.

— Chew young leaf shoots of the silver birch or swallow these in great quantities to aid digestion, prevent constipation or cure constipation. It also helps to promote a clear complexion.

— Eat linseeds daily.

— Take fresh sea tangle, cut in pieces and chew. Then swallow.

— Take the root of buckbean. Clean and boil it in water all day until the juice is dark and thick. Strain this and take only a teaspoonful as it is very strong.

— Eat soaked prunes for breakfast.

Cramps

— Take a hip bath lasting for one half hour, using water as

hot as possible.

— Take half an ounce of: ointment of marsh-mallows; oil of worms; two drachms of oil of turpentine; two scruples of camphire; two drachms of compound spirit of lavender; six drops of oil of cloves. Make a liniment and oil the affected part well with a warm hand.

— To cure cramps in the legs, take the last pair of shoes you were wearing and if the cramp is in the left leg, take the left shoe and put it inside the right shoe and place them under the bed for a week. Do the opposite for cramp in the right leg.

— Grandmother's remedy for cramp that makes the sufferer leap out of bed was to have a piece of cork handy to rub on the affected part. This was said to stop the cramp immediately.

— Place a magnet under the pillow if suffering from night-cramp and it will not return.

Croup

— Old Dutch remedy: Equal quantities of goose oil and urine. Dose: from one teaspoon to a tablespoon of the mixture according to the age of the child. Repeat the dose every fifteen minutes till the child vomits.

— A piece of fresh lard, as large as a butternut, rubbed up with sugar, in the same way that butter and sugar are prepared for the dressing of puddings, divided into three parts. One part taken every twenty minutes will relieve any case of croup if it has not already been allowed to progress to the fatal point.

Deafness

— Take clean, fine black wool, dip it in civet and put it into the ear. When it dries out in a day or two, dip it in again and

keep the wool moist in the ear for three weeks or a month.
— Griddle the fat from the kidneys of wild rabbit and put two drops in each ear every night. Rub cotton wool to a point, dip it in the kidney fat and put it in the ear. Let it remain till hearing improves.

Diarrhoea

— Drink a mixture of raw oats. Eat plenty of cooked brown rice with bilberries.
— Eat oatmeal gruel daily.
— Drink tormentilla tea daily.
— Coffee charcoal is very useful in cases of diarrhoea.
— Eat a peeled and grated apple.
— Drink only black tea and eat toasted white bread with cinnamon only.
— Eat boiled bleached rice with cinnamon.
— Remove the moss from trees, boil it in red wine and drink it.
— Chronic diarrhoea is cured by drinking orange peel tea, sweetened with loaf-sugar, used as a common drink for twenty-four or thirty-six hours.
— Every hour take a tablespoon of aromatic syrup of rhubarb till the diarrhoea is checked.

Earache

— Use onion poultices.
— Put a few drops of heated St John's wort oil in the ear.
— Put a clove of garlic in the ear or a small toasted fig and bathe the feet in warm water at bedtime. Take care to cover the ear with some cotton wool and keep the head warm during the night.
— Take a bit of cotton batting, put upon it a pinch of black

pepper, gather it up and tie it. Dip it in sweet oil and insert it into the ear. Put a flannel bandage on the head to keep it warm.

— Take the juice of mountain sage, oil of fennel, or oil of olives, and mix well together; drop into the pained ear three drops for several nights.

— To kill earwigs or other insects in the ear: Let the person under this distressing circumstance lay his head upon the table, the side upwards that is afflicted: at the same time let some friend carefully drop into the ear some sweet oil or oil of almonds. A drop or two will be sufficient to instantly destroy the insect and remove the pain, however violent.

— Indian cure for earache: Take a piece of lean mutton, the size of a large walnut, put it into the fire and burn it for some time till it is reduced to a cinder. Then put it into a piece of clean cloth and squeeze it until some moisture is extracted which must be dropped into the ear as hot as the patient can stand it.

— Take a large onion and slice it. Then cut strong tobacco leaves to the same size. Alternately place a tobacco leaf and an onion slice on top of each other. Wrap this into a wet cloth and cover in hot embers until the onion is cooked. Press out the juice with heavy pressure and drop the juice into the ear.

— Place a limpet on the fire and remove when the juice bubbles. When cooled down slightly, pour the juice into the ear and stop the ear with a bit of sheep's wool that still contains the natural oil.

Eczema

— Follow a cleansing diet of carrot, beetroot and parsley.
— Follow a juice diet and use a good laxative.

— Green vegetable juices are important for the supply of chlorophyll to eczema patients.

— Dab afflicted areas with milk whey.

— Use a herbal mixture of dandelions, comfrey, periwinkle and golden seal on the affected area.

— Drink goat's milk instead of cow's milk.

— Take oil of evening-primrose.

Emphysema

— Use a poultice of horsetail overnight.

— Drink Irish moss tea.

— Use garlic every day.

Eyes

— For eyes that are red and sore: Take a red cabbage leaf and bruise it, then mix it with the white of an egg. Cover the eyes with this mixture and leave it on all night.

— Add a decoction of elder flowers and three or four drops of laudanum to a small glass of tea. Let the mixture run into the eye three or four times daily. A cure is effected in one week.

— Mix one dram of salt of tartar with a pint of frog's spawn. Let them dissolve together and anoint the eyes with this mixture several times daily.

— Stye upon the eye-lid: Put a teaspoon of black tea in a small bag and pour on enough water to moisten it. While still pretty warm, place the bag on the eye. Keep it on all night with a bandage and in the morning the stye will most likely be gone. If not, a second application is certain to remove it. Nowadays a tea bag could be used.

— To recover or strengthen weak eyesight: Take half an ounce each of cloves and nutmeg; two pennies worth of

English saffron, a handful of eye-bright leaves dried in the sun, and make all these into a fine powder. Then take eight or nine raisins, stone them, and put in them as much powder as will lie on a penny. Eat them in the morning and do not eat anything else for the first hour after having eaten these raisins.

— Inflammation of the eyes: Mix bread crumbs with the white of an egg, three drops of brandy and very little salt. Apply in a bag of thin soft linen or muslin. It is better to apply it at night when lying down. Also drink eye-bright tea and wash the eyes with it.

— Boil some eye-bright leaves in water, cool and sieve it. Use this extract to bathe the eyes with when irritated and tired.

— For weak eyes: A concoction of the flowers of daisies boiled down is an excellent eye-wash, to be used constantly.

— Place used cool camomile tea bags on the eyes.

— Potato poultice: Grate the potato finely and strain some of the juice onto a cotton wool pad. Place the pad gently on the affected and inflamed eye.

— For brighter eyes: Weigh out equal quantities of rose petals, cornflowers and camomile flowers. Mix and boil them in water for five minutes. Sieve and cool and then place the flowers between pieces of gauze. Place a compress over each of your eye-lids for ten minutes each morning and evening.

— For tired eyes: Boil some cornflowers in water. Allow them to cool after straining and put the flowers between layers of gauze. Lie flat for fifteen minutes and place a compress over each eye.

— To soothe swollen eye-lids: Apply raw potato cut in slices each morning and evening.

— Eye inflammation: Make a poultice of beaten egg white and place on the eye.

— For a stye: Point a sharp steel instrument at the stye while reciting a Gaelic incantation.

— Boil birds foot trefoil in water and use as eye-wash.

— Infuse eye-bright in either water or milk to bathe the eyes.

— Rub with pure gold.

— Wash with freshly made tea which has cooled.

— Take the small white bones found in the head of a haddock, one behind each eye. Powder these into dust and apply to the stye. This will cure it.

Fever

— To break a fever catch a granddaddy spider, pull its legs off and swallow it whole and alive.

— Drink holly tea mixed with goldenrod.

— Use onion and vinegar compresses on the stomach.

— Drink plenty of fluids, especially barley water.

Foot Problems

— Take house leeks, bruise them and apply to corns on the feet. This will cure them.

— Take nightshade berries, boil them in hog's lard and anoint the corn with the salve. It will not fail to cure.

— Blisters on the feet due to much walking can be cured by drawing a needleful of worsted thread through them. Clip it off at both ends and leave until the skin peels off.

— When suffering from cold feet, rub some St John's wort oil in.

— Oil for aching feet: Mix together five tablespoons of sesame oil and five drops of clove oil. Massage well into the feet.

TRADITIONAL HOME AND HERBAL REMEDIES

Freckles and Pimples

— Bitter almonds and barley flour, in equal parts, applied in the form of a paste will remove freckles.

— Two fluid ounces of thick barleywater. Two fluid ounces of distilled water of bean-flowers. Two fluid ounces spirits of wine. Wash the freckled or tanned skin frequently with this preparation.

— Bathe the face in morning dew.

— Anoint a freckled face with the blood of a bull, or of a hare, and it will remove the freckles and make the skin fair and clear. The distilled water of walnuts is also effective.

— Grate horseradish finely, let it stand for a few hours in buttermilk, then strain and use the wash morning and night.

— Squeeze the juice of a lemon into half a goblet of water and use this to wash the affected areas every night and morning.

— Remedy for pimples: Take half a quarter of a pound of bitter almonds, blanch and pulverise them and put them into half a pint of spring water. Mix together and strain, add to half a pint of the best brandy and a pennyworth of the best brimstone. Shake it well and frequently dab it on with a soft cloth.

Gallstones

— Drink horseradish tea.

— A very good, though drastic cure is the lemon and olive oil cure: one pint of olive oil and half a pint of lemon juice mixed. Start at seven p.m. and then use equal amounts every fifteen minutes. Fast all day before starting this course.

— Another oil cure for gallstones. If the person suffering from gallstones is able to drink half a pint of oil at one time, then the oil cure should be considered before any surgical operation to remove gallstones. The oil does not enter the gallbladder, but merely stimulates the secretion of bile which will carry the small and medium stones with it. Olive oil should be used for this purpose. Artichokes and other herbal remedies should be taken before starting this oil cure in order to liquify the gall. As the bowels should be cleansed well, it is recommended to eat soaked prunes or figs. If this does not bring the required effect, an enema of warm water with camomile should be used. When the bowels are empty the half pint of oil can be drunk and hot packs should be placed on the liver area two hours before and two hours after drinking the oil.

Lie down on the right side for two hours. If not able to drink the oil by itself, it may be mixed with coffee or it may be drunk at intervals. This will be less effective, but will still cleanse the liver and smaller stones will still come away, although the bigger stones are left behind. These, however, may not be too bothersome for a period of time. If capable of drinking the oil all at one time, the bigger stones may also be flushed away. If the situation has become chronic, surgery might be the only answer. As the oil cure has proved satisfactory in many cases, there is little doubt that this method is much preferable to surgery, which undoubtedly has after-effects.

Gout

— Chew grains of mustard seeds daily.
— Rub the affected part with warm treacle and then bind on a flannel smeared with this. If necessary, repeat this action every twelve hours. It has cured bad cases of gout in thirty-six hours.
— Drink a pint of strong infusion of elder buds, dry or green, morning and evening.

— At six in the evening, undress and wrap yourself in blankets. Put your legs up to the knees in water, as hot as you are able to endure it. As the water cools, pour in more hot water so as to keep you in a strong sweat till ten. Go to bed well warmed and sweat till morning.

— Take the oldest tallow you can get and garlic, in equal parts. Stamp them together, spread it on canvas and lay it on the affected parts. It eases the pain.

— Take rendered goat's milk, butter and add roast cow's manure. Mix and apply to a cloth which should be placed on the sore areas.

Haemorrhoids

— Use yarrow extract externally.
— Sponge the affected area with ice cold water.
— A mixture of tormentilla and nettles will help.

Hair

— Daily drink tea made from the stinging nettle, walnut leaves and elder leaves when losing hair.

— Brandy and salt are supposed to have the power of restoring hair, though sheep dip was considered better in the outback of Australia.

— Boil the roots of the elm for a long time in water, and clean scum off the fat arising at the top. Anoint the place that is grown bald, and the hair fallen away will quickly restore them again.

— Rub the bald part frequently with the juice of an onion until it looks red.

— Mix one pint of water, half an ounce of pearlash, a quarter pint of onion juice, one-eighth of a pint of rum and twenty drops of oil of rosemary. Rub the head hard with a rough linen towel dipped in this mixture.

— Make an infusion of one and three-quarter ounces of nettle leaves of the small variety of nettle in one and three-quarter pints of vinegar. Warm the vinegar before adding the leaves and leave it to soak for half an hour. Strain and use the tea as a lotion for massaging the scalp.

— Take three and a half ounces of roots of burdock and two ounces of small nettle leaves. Chop and marinate in four-fifths of a pint of rum for at least one week and strain through some fine linen.

Take three and a half ounces each of nasturtium, nettle and box leaves and chop them finely. Marinate in four-fifths of a pint of rum for two weeks. Strain and use as lotion for the scalp.

— As a hair softener the yoghurt treatment may be used. After washing and handtowelling the hair spread thick yoghurt all over. Leave for ten minutes and rinse off with lukewarm water.

— Soft hair can be given some body if the last rinse is done with beer.

— Make camomile tea and use this as the last rinse after washing the hair to obtain a nice gloss (particularly suitable for blond hair). This also has the effect that the hair does not go greasy too soon.

— To lighten the hair: Use the juice of a lemon for the last rinse and let the hair dry in the sunshine.

Hayfever

— Drink stinging nettle tea.
— Use bee pollens.
— Eat honey daily.
— Packs of Epsom salt and grapefruit over the face will bring relief.

TRADITIONAL HOME AND HERBAL REMEDIES

Headache

— Wet coarse brown paper with strong cider vinegar and place on the forehead. Also bathe the eyes in cold water.

— Take marigold flowers and distill them. Take a fine cloth and wet it with the distilled water. Place it on the forehead and try to sleep.

— Take goat's dung and mix it with vinegar of squills. Anoint the head and temple herewith.

— Beat an egg together with frankincense and myrrh and apply this to the head and temples.

— Two ounces of rhubarb, sliced. One ounce of powdered jesuit's bark. Two ounces of sugar candy. Two drams of juniper berries. One dram each of cinnamon and nutmeg. One quart of wine. Infuse these together and apply to the head.

— Use onion and cabbage poultices on the neck.

— Place cold compresses on forehead and refresh frequently.

— Boil the leaves of the buckbean and drink the water first thing in the morning. Gather the entire plant, dry it, boil and drink the juice for a severe headache.

— Place a horseradish poultice on the nape of the neck.

Hiccups

— Put as much dill seed, finely powdered, as will lie on a shilling, into two spoonfuls of black cherries and take it immediately.

— For prevention of hiccups: Infuse a scruple of musk in a quart of mountain wine and take a small glass every morning.

— Tickle your nose with a feather to induce a sneeze.

— Drink in one draught a large glass of water in which

there is an eggspoon. Drain the glass to the last drop.
— Take a pinch of snuff to make you sneeze.
— Swallow half an ice cube.
— Ask someone to give you a fright — e.g. by suddenly slapping you on the back.
— Hold your breath while mentally counting slowly to twenty.
— Breathe in and out of a paper bag twenty times.
— Drink a glass of water from the opposite side of the glass.

Hoarseness

— Chew rowanberries and pimpernel well.
— Use warm, moist throat poultices.

Indigestion

— Two tablespoons of bicarbonate of soda mixed with one teaspoon of ground ginger. Take one teaspoonful in hot water before breakfast.
— To cure heartburn a teacup full of camomile tea, or a small quantity of chalk scraped into a glass of water, are deemed effectual remedies.
— Acid stomach: Take good unslaked lime, the quarter of the size of a hen's egg to one pint of soft water. Strain and keep cool. Take one teaspoon to half a cup of fresh milk each morning and night.
— Drink a pint of cold water.
— Slowly drink camomile tea.
— Eat four or five oysters.
— Slightly chew five or six peppercorns and then swallow them.
— Chew fennel or parsley and then swallow your spittle.

— Chew a piece of Spanish liquorice.
— Use oil of peppermint.
— Place an onion poultice on the stomach.
— Take a hot shower.
— Use a cabbage poultice on the stomach area.

Insomnia

— Drink an extract of oats before retiring.
— Wash the head in a decoction of dill seed and smell it frequently.
— If you go to sleep lying flat on your back, you will not have a nightmare. A cure for nightmares is found by turning the shoes upside down with the toes towards the head of the bed.
— To prevent a nightmare: Avoid heavy suppers, and on going to bed take a mixture of twenty drops of sal volatile and two drachms of ginger.
— To induce sleep use lemon balm.

Jaundice

— Tie up equal parts of soot and saffron in a piece of cloth. Let it lie in a glass of water overnight. In the morning beat the yolk of an egg, add this to the water and drink it. Do this three mornings, then skipping three, etc, until nine doses have been taken.
— Take as much carrot juice as possible. Sprinkle salads with dandelion.
— Hot showers on the liver area and use hot herb compresses.
— Do not use any fats.
— Make and drink barley water: use three-quarters of a gallon of water to one cup of barley.

— Take a bath to which plenty of Epsom salt has been added.
— Jaundice is got by fright and must be cured by a fright. He who drinks the first milk of the cow after calving will never take jaundice.

Kidneys

— Daily drink the tea of the following mixture: horsetail, shepherd's purse and birch leaves.
— Every morning take a teaspoonful of glycerine on an empty stomach for kidney stones.
— Drink potato water frequently.
— Drink four cups of peach leaf tea daily.
— Beet tops and beetroots will dissolve kidney stones.

Lumbago

— To effect a cure have someone who was born feet first stand on your back.

Mumps

— Wrap the child in a blanket, take it to the pigsty, rub the child's head on the back of a pig and the mumps will leave it and pass from the child to the animal.
— Take a hip bath and make sure the water temperature is between 97° and 110°F.
— Use warm compresses of arnica or marigold.
— Apply locally, warm St John's wort oil compresses.

Nerves

— Every day eat porridge or oats.
— Use valerian herbs.

— Place some hop herbs into the pillow.

Night sweats

— Daily drink sage tea.
— Infuse a tea from mixed lady's-mantle and horsetail and drink daily.

Nosebleeds

— To prevent nosebleeds: Drink milk whey every morning and eat plenty of raisins. Or, dissolve two scruples of nitre in half a pint of water and take a teacupful every hour.
— To cure nosebleeds:
Apply to the neck behind and on each side, a cloth dipped in cold water.
Or, put the legs and arms in cold water.
Or, wash the temples, nose and neck with vinegar.
Or, keep a little roll of white paper under the tongue.
Or, snuff up vinegar and water.
Or, foment the legs with it.
Or, steep a linen cloth in sharp vinegar, burn it and blow up the nose with a quill.
Or, apply tents made of soft linen dipped in cold water, strongly impregnated with tincture of iron and introduced within the nostrils quite through to their posterior apertures.
In a violent case, go into a pond or river.
(from Rev John Wesley's *Primitive Physick*, 1747)
— Crowd the fingers tight into the ears and, pressing the teeth well together, act as if chewing food.
— Bend the head forward and place a cold metal key in the back of the neck.

Psoriasis

— Follow a diet consisting solely of raw foods. First a fast of seven days using only water. Then a diet of fruit juice, nuts, maize bread, raw salads and potatoes.
— Drink Solidago — Goldenrod tea.
— Drink the tea made of willow bark, stinging nettle, oak bark, calendula and yarrow.
— Dab nettle extract onto the affected psoriasis parts.
— Drink milk whey daily.

Rheumatism

— For chronic rheumatism take two ounces each of skunk oil and cheap lamp oil and one teaspoon of red pepper. Shake well together and bathe the affected parts with a piece of flannel dipped into this mixture.
— Boil two potatoes in their jackets. When done, mash potatoes, skins and all, spread on a cloth and apply.
— A successful recipe from an old Indian squaw: A large kettle is filled with water which is thickened to a poultice consistency with chopped red peppers and the mixture is boiled for an hour or so. Into this a linen sheet is dropped and placed, steaming hot, about the body of the patient. In the meantime, blankets have been heated and with them a veritable inferno-bed prepared into which the patient is tightly tucked and fed cup after cup of hot tea until he sweats the rheumatism out of his system.
— Chew two or three juniper berries daily.
— Always carry a nutmeg or potato in the pocket.
— Boil sea water and put it on the sore joints as hot as can be borne. Put sulphur in the soles of the stockings.
— Take half a pound each of prickly ash berries, spikenard root, yellow poplar and dogwood barks. Pulverise and put

into a gallon jug and fill it with brandy. Dose: a wine glass of it is to be taken three times daily before meals.

Ringworm

— Put milk whey in the bath water.
— Dab with milk whey or Molkosan.

Shingles

— Soothe affected parts with the juice of fresh leeks.
— Drink daily three cups full of tea made from the following herbs:
    20 gram camomile
    20 gram lady's-mantle
    20 gram melilot
    20 gram solidago
    30 gram oak bark
    30 gram of oats
    30 gram sage
    30 gram valerian
— Cut up three ounces of garlic and simmer in water for about five minutes. Add three ounces of sulphur, one ounce of saltpetre, two ounces of liquorice, two tablespoons of water and two tablespoons of vinegar. Simmer for a further five minutes. Leave till dissolved, strain and bottle. Take one tablespoon last thing at night and first thing in the morning.

Skin problems

— To make a swarthy complexion appear agreeable: Sift the flour out of half a peck of wheatbran, then crack into the bran eight newly laid eggs, and six pints of white wine vinegar. Let the eggs be beaten well and when these ingredients are properly mixed, let it distill over a slow fire.

When it has stood for a day to settle, take a little of it and rub your face every day for a fortnight and it will look extremely fair.

— Make a hole in a lemon, fill it with sugar candy and close it nicely with leaf gold applied over the rind where it was cut. Then roast the lemon in hot ashes. Squeeze some of the juice through the hole and wash the face with a napkin wetted thus. This juice greatly cleanses the skin and brightens up the complexion.

— To smooth the skin of the hands: twenty grams of almond oil, thirty grams of pure glycerin, fifty grams of lemon juice and twenty grams of eau de cologne. Shake these ingredients in a bottle and several times daily massage a small amount into the hands.

— Four dessertspoons of almond oil, four dessertspoons of peachstone oil and one and a half teaspoons of bees wax. Mix both oils, then melt the bees wax over some hot water and add to the mixed oils. The result will be an ideal cream to soften the skin of the hands.

— If suffering from red hands: Boil one litre of water with one hundred grams of sea salt. Cool this down slightly so that it is still hot, but bearable. Immerse both hands into this and keep them there for twenty minutes.

— Chapped hands: Make a paste of one hundred grams of castor oil, five grams of bergamot oil, five grams of mint oil and five grams of pure camphor. Starting in autumn this paste should be used on the hands daily to prevent chapped skin in winter.

— Brandy and cucumber hand lotion: two tablespoonfuls of cucumber, peeled and mashed. Two tablespoonfuls of glycerine, two tablespoonfuls of brandy, two tablespoonfuls of rosewater. Whisk all the ingredients together, pot and store. Use to your liking.

Snake bites

— Viper or rattlesnake bite: Apply bruised garlic. Or, rub the place with common oil.

— Rattlesnake bites: An old physician was called to a boy who was bitten by a rattlesnake. In the absence of any other remedies, he cured the boy on the principle of "the hair of the dog will cure his bite". He took a piece of the snake about two inches long, split it on the back and bound it onto the bite. It cleansed the wound and no bad effects were seen from it.

— Wet carbonate of soda should be applied externally to the bite of a spider or any venomous creature and it will neutralise the poisonous effects almost immediately. It acts like a charm in the case of a snake bite.

— Lean fresh meat will remove the pain of a wasp sting almost instantly and has been recommended for the cure of rattlesnake bites.

Splinters

— To remove a splinter, take boiling lard or fat and either put this on with a limpet shell or dip the finger into the hot fat. Lard or fat are preferable to butter, as they hold greater heat.

Sprains and Strains

— Beat an egg white, spread it on a piece of linen and bandage this poultice onto the sprained area. Leave it on until the egg white has hardened. It is also good to add some camphor powder to the egg white while beating.

— Apply a plaster of chopped parsley mixed with butter.

— Rub gently with a piece of rag or wool dipped in olive oil and cover with a compress saturated with the oil. Sprains will soon heal.

— Immediately apply a cloth folded five or six times, dipped in cold water and refresh frequently.

— Spread molasses on brown paper and apply immediately to the affected area.

— Take a spoonful of honey, the same quantity of salt, and the white of an egg. Beat these together and anoint the sprained area with this, keeping it well rolled in a good bandage.

— Skin an eel in long strips and wrap it round as a bandage with the fat side in. The eel fat soothes the skin and, as it is elastic, will not bind it too tightly.

— Rub the strain in a running stream.

Stings

— Salt and vinegar is a valuable remedy for the sting of a bee. Wet the salt with vinegar and lay it on in the form of a poultice. It will extract the sting. If stung on the hand or some other accessible part, instantly apply the mouth to the wound, draw it powerfully till some other remedy is provided.

— Sand flea bites should be dabbed with some cotton wool soaked in petrol. In case no petrol is available some wet tobacco also seems to ease the discomfort.

— To ward off midges or mosquitos take some buttercups and rub these over the exposed areas. Make sure to break the flowers and stems on the skin.

— During the summer season when midges are about use extra garlic in the preparation of your salads and other foods. This will keep midges away.

— A simple and effective cure for those who may accidentally have swallowed a wasp: Instantly on the alarming accident taking place, put a teaspoon of common salt in your mouth. This will not only kill the wasp instantaneously, but at the same time heal the sting.

Stomach problems

— Drink the water in which onions have been boiled.
— Take half a sheet of cap-paper, cut it in the shape of a heart and dip it in equal quantities of brandy and candle grease, mixed together. Apply it warm to the pit of the stomach.
— Warm water sweetened with molasses or warm sugar, taken freely, will often remove the cramp in the stomach when opium and other medicines have failed.
— When a patient is in desperation put a rope round his feet and hang him by the heels from the rafters. Repeat at reasonable intervals. This will undo the knot in the guts.
— Indigestion: Take fresh dulse from the seashore and eat it raw.
— Carrageen boiled in either milk or water is very soothing to a sore stomach.
— Boil the entire plant of tormentil and drink the juice.
— Boil nettle tops and drink the juice.

Stomach ulcers

— Boil the roots of bogbeans and, when cooled, drink the juice obtained for stomach ailments.
— Chew the raw roots of tobacco for stomach complaints.
— To aid digestion after a heavy meal, drink the infusion of sage, a few leaves in a cup of boiling water. Or put a pinch of aniseed in some warm water and drink this.
— Every day eat a raw grated potato or extract the juice

from a raw potato and drink that.

Teething problems

— Boil poppy flowers with sugar and water. Give the baby one teaspoon of this extract at night. This has an opium effect.

— Use camomile extract on the gums.

Toothache

— Wash the root of an aching tooth in elder vinegar and let it dry in the sun for half an hour.

— Split a raisin and put a little mustard on the sticky side and apply to the aching tooth or gum. It will draw out all the soreness.

— Boil a raisin or a small fig in milk and apply to the tooth while hot.

— One quarter pound of pale Peruvian bark, finely powdered. One pint of old four proof French brandy. One pint of rosewater. One pint of pure water. Mix and after twenty four hours it is fit for use. For severe toothache, add more brandy in one to four proportion to the above and hold this concoction in the mouth for at least five minutes.

— Fill a small bag with heated salt and place on the painful area.

— Mix gunpowder and tallow and put it into the cavity, chewing it in.

— Fill the cavity with archangel tar.

— Make a poultice of archangel tar in a piece of linen and plaster the cheek with it.

— Carry in your pocket the two jaw-bones of a haddock; for ever since the miracle of the loaves and fishes these bones are an infallible remedy against toothache. The older the bones are the better, as they are nearer the time of the miracle.

— Take two garlic perles every two hours.

Varicose Ulcers – Open

— Use clay poultices.

— Make a poultice of equal amounts of cod liver oil and honey and bandage a poultice in place overnight.

— If fresh Russian comfrey is available, grate it and place on the leg with a clay poultice.

— Place a cabbage-leaf poultice on the affected area.

— Use mustard flour poultices.

Vomiting

— Take a large nutmeg and grate away half of it. Toast the flat side till the oil oozes out. Then clap it to the pit of the stomach. Let it lie so long as it is warm. Repeat till the problem is cured.

— For vomiting and diarrhoea: Take pulverised cloves and eat them together with bread soaked in red wine and you will soon find relief. The cloves may be put on bread.

— Cut a large onion and apply to the pit of the stomach.

— Use a spoonful of lemon juice and six grains of salt of wormwood.

Warts

— Make a white turnip hollow by taking the pit out. In the hollow put fresh butter and a fresh hen's egg. Let these articles be rendered by broiling inside. Pour through a cloth, with a little rosewater added, and boil it till it becomes the consistency of a salve. Very reliable for the treatment of warts.

— Cut a piece of wild turnip, from the woods, and rub several times upon the wart.

— Rub warts with fig leaves and bury the said leaves in the earth. The warts will go away as the leaves rot.

— Rub warts with the inside of a broad bean and afterwards throw the broad bean away.

— Rub warts daily with a radish, or with marigold flowers. This will hardly fail.

— Find a black slug and rub the wart with it.

— Rub the wart with radish juice or sloeberry juice twice a day until the wart disappears.

— Put nine of the joints of the corn (oats) in a hidden place, such as under a stone. Do not go near them again and as they wear away the warts will also disappear.

— Daily rub the wart with garlic juice.

— Soak lemon peel for two weeks in vinegar and then place the lemon peel onto the wart and bandage it.

— Daily bathe warts with water in which sal ammoniac has been dissolved.

— Apply to the wart a poultice of bruised purslain, changing it twice daily.

— Rub daily with dandelions.

— Common salt used for itch etc, also clears warts. Wet the wart, sprinkle salt over it and cover it with a small bandage.

— Roast chicken feet and rub the warts with them and then bury the chicken feet under the eaves.

— Use Chelidonium tea daily.

Water Treatments

— In Scotland it was believed that extraordinary curative properties were to be found in wells. The patient drank the water and bathed in it. The St Ninian's Well in Prestwick was used by Robert The Bruce and is said to have cured him of leprosy.

— Father Kneipp recommended lightning-fast water treatments for only a few seconds on various parts of the body. The water should be at room temperature and not ice-cold and the body as warm as possible. The whole body should be wetted quickly and the skin should not be rubbed dry. Instead press the water gently into the pores with a sponge or damp towel. As soon as this action is finished one should get dressed and take some exercise to regain body heat. According to Father Kneipp blood obstructions are the main cause of disease. "When these obstructions occur in various parts of the body, the blood remains cooped up, neither able to advance or retard properly." The principle behind his recommendations is simple: water temperature affects circulation, either to increase or reduce it. This is especially important when tissues or organs are congested or inflamed.

— In China the following methods are recommended:

The drinking of six large tumblers of water at one time renders the colon more effective in forming more new fresh blood. This is made possible by the function of neucosa folds found in the nutrients from food taken by our bodies. They are turned into fresh blood. This theory was published in an article written by a Japanese professor some years ago.

Due to insufficient exercise of the colonic tract, man feels exhausted and becomes sick. Adults have colons or large intestines eight feet long and capable of absorbing the nutrients taken several times a day. If the colon is clean, then the nutrients taken will be completely absorbed by the neucosa fold which will turn them into new fresh blood.

This blood is responsible for curing our ailments and is considered as a prime power in the improvement of our health. In other words the "Water Therapy" will make us healthy and prolong our mortal lives.

A sick person might find it difficult to drink large quantities of water, but should persevere. Wherever possible try to take exercise after the drinking of the water.

Bedridden people who are unable to get up and do some exercises after drinking the water should practice deep inspiration and expiration while lying in bed and massage their stomachs with the purpose of making the water inside the colon flow so as to wash and clean the neucosa folds. Some people will experience loose bowels and may have to urinate maybe as much as three times in one hour. However, after three or four days, the trouble will be eliminated.

When suffering from gastritis, a cure will be affected in one week by using the water treatment. Older people suffering from arthritis and rheumatism should undergo water therapy three times a day for one week.

Weakness

— If suffering from general weakness make a tea of the following: Agrimony, ripple grass (rib grass), red nettles, aniseed, sage and parsley. Daily drink this tea till improvement is experienced.

Whooping cough

— It is said that physicians in Paris have discovered a definite cure for whooping cough. The suffering child is sent to a neighbouring gas factory to inhale for a few minutes the vapours which arise from the lime used to purify gas. Two or three visits effect a radical cure.

— One gill each of onions and garlic, sliced. One gill of sweet oil. Stew the vegetables in the oil in a covered dish to obtain the juices. Strain and add one gill of honey. Add half an ounce each of paregoric and spirits of camphor. Bottle and cork. Dose: for children of two to three years old, one teaspoon three or four times daily or, when the cough is troublesome, increasing or lessening according to age.

— Cut three small bunches of hair from the crown of the head of the child that has never seen its father. Sew this hair in an unbleached rag and hang it round the neck of the child suffering from whooping cough. The thread with which the sack is sewn should also be unbleached.

— Thrust the child with whooping cough three times through a blackberry bush without speaking or saying anything. The bush, however, must be grown fast at the two ends, and the child must be thrust through three times in the same manner, that is to say, from the same place it was thrust through in the first place.

— The very best thing for whooping cough is to drink mare's milk.

— Make a syrup of prickly pear and drink freely. Take three moderate-sized leaves of the prickly pear to a quart of cold water, cut up in pieces and boil slowly for about half an hour. Strain out all the prickles through some muslin, sweeten with white sugar and boil a bit longer.

Worms

— Pare bog myrtle. Boil in water to make strong drink and take after fasting.

— Salt herrings fried on red cinders should be eaten after fasting. Then in an hour or two drink as much water as possible.
— Use plant of garlic.

Wounds

— Apply horseradish poultices.
— Dab with diluted whey or Molkosan.
— Use cabbage poultices.

Wry neck – Torticollis

— Use plenty of garlic internally and externally.

Cures for animals

— Red water in cows: Boil the entire plant of the pansy. Put the juice in a bottle and pour down the cow's throat.
— Dry disease in cows:
Boil bracken roots and make the cow drink the juice.
Or, press some small white whelks and place them in a bottle of cold water. Feed this to the cow daily.
Or, feed the cow daily a handful of black slugs without shells.
Or, boil seaweed in water and feed the water as well as the weed to the cow daily.
— Constipation in cows:
For constipation in calves the buckbean should be used. One glassful of liquid is sufficient. A handful of white whelks pounded fine, should be given to the cows every morning. Alternatively collect the tiniest, white whelks and keep them in buckets of salt water to keep them alive. If fed alive to a constipated cow, they are said to break up the mass and enable bowel movements. They are also said to cure any obstruction, i.e. growth, in the digestive system as they would eat the growth away.

TRADITIONAL HOME AND HERBAL REMEDIES

— Colds in cows: Give the cow some hot milk to drink with plenty of pepper in it.

— Cataract in cows and sheep: Pound glass to a fine powder and put it in the eye of the animal, covering it with a shield and it will wear away.

— Staggers: To cure a horse of staggers, cut a vein below the right ear and let so much blood away.

— Tonic for coughs and colds: Administer one pint of seal oil at a time.

— Lump in the throat: This disease is found particularly in sheep. Take a turf from the roof of a thatched house and set it alight. Keep the sheep's face over it so that it will inhale the smoke until the nose and mouth water plentifully. This is said to be a complete cure.

— Lump on a horse: Cut it out and apply to the open wound for several days a salt and water pickle, so strong that a potato will float in it.

— Diarrhoea in dogs: Dogs with diarrhoea may be so weak that they are unable to get to their feet. Even veterinarian's prescriptions may fail. Feed the dog with steamed onions and garlic perles and steamed carrots.

— Worms in dogs: Daily add several garlic perles or fresh garlic and steamed onions to the dog's food. It may take two or three weeks before all the worms and eggs have been removed.

— Eczema in dogs: This causes a lot of discomfort for dogs. They will scratch and bite until raw spots appear. It is advisable to prevent eczema by supplementing their rations with bone meal, flax seed, steamed onions and carrots, Vitamin C complex, garlic perles and chlorophyll perles.

— Pink-eye in dogs: This is a contagious epidemic conjunctivitis. Hot packs of Lipton's tea over the eyes and drops of Lipton's tea in the eyes will relieve the inflammation. Healing will be assisted by administering one hundred milligrams of Vitamin C and some chlorophyll and garlic perles every hour. Onion poultices over the eyes will also help. Onions should be steamed in a pan, thickened with flax seed meal and applied over the eyes in a sack. The poultice should be kept warm.

— Flea repellent: It is unnecessary and sometimes even fatal to use poison sprays, powders and collars on pets. B1 is an excellent flea repellent. Pets lose their fleas when fed yeast and liver regularly. These are good sources of B1.

— For a fine coat of hair: If daily some wheat germ is mixed with the food or some wheat germ oil is given pets will produce a healthy, shiny coat of hair.

Friends, doctors, patients, farmers and shepherds have helped me to compile this colourful collection of home remedies from which I have been forced to make a selection. I am grateful to my gardeners who have helped me with information regarding the growing and planting. I am also grateful to the doctor's widow from South Uist, who visited the older inhabitants on the island and noted down many old remedies, and to the retired rector of one of the local high schools. So many people made it possible for me to collect this information.

An ancient Chinese aphorism states: "The further back we look, the further forward we may see." With this in mind I express the hope that this book may be a source of help in relieving some of the aches, pains, problems and ailments with which our society is plagued.

Bibliography and Literature

Vogel A — *The Nature Doctor* (eighth edition), 1977, Verlag A Vogel, Teufen AR, Switzerland.

Comrie, John D, MA, BSc, MD, FRCP — *History of Scottish Medicine to 1860* Wellcome Historical Medical Museum, by Bailliere Tindall and Cox, London.

Nicholas Culpeper — *Culpeper's Complete Herbal,* W Foulsham and Co Ltd, London.

Peter Tomkins and Christopher Bird — *The Secret Life of Plants* The Trinity Press, Ebenezer Bayliss and Son Ltd, Worcester and London.

The Language of Flowers, Ballantyne Press, Frederick Warne and Co, London.

Jean Palaiseul — *Grandmother's Secrets*, First edition 1973, Barrie and Jenkins, Penguin Books Ltd, Harmondsworth, Middlesex.

British Herbal Pharmacopoeia. Part One 1976. British Herbal Medicine Association, London WC1.

Daems W F — *Geneeskruiden'. Deel 1,* C V Uitgeverij Tittera

Scripta Manet, Naarden, Holland.

Mellie Uyldert — *Lexicon der Geneeskruiden*, Uitgeverij De Driehoek, Amsterdam.

Carol Bishop — *The Book of Home Remedies and Herbal Cures*, Octopus Books Ltd, London W1.

Magdea Ironside Wood — *Herbs*, Marshall Cavendish Books Ltd, London W1.